"Whether you are an exasperated or apprehensive parent of a picky eater or you just want to be a better parent, you need this resource. With wisdom, wit, and candor, Dr. Nimali Fernando and Melanie Potock take you on a fascinating journey into the mind and sensory system of your fickle eaters."

—DANIEL FEITEN, MD, clinical professor of pediatrics, University of Colorado School of Medicine founder and CEO, Pediatric Web Inc. and RemedyConnect Inc.

"Dr. Nimali Fernando and Melanie Potock offer exceptional, timeless advice on how to create an eating environment that is healthy, happy, and stress-free for child and parent. A very difficult task, but they have hit a home run with this book."

—THEODORE STATHOS, MD, professor of pediatrics, Rocky Vista University College of Osteopathic Medicine, director of pediatric gastroenterology and nutrition, The Rocky Mountain Hospital for Children, president, Rocky Mountain Pediatric Gastroenterology

"Dr. Nimali Fernando and Melanie Potock provide innovative, fun, healthy, and, most importantly, doable solutions to just about every challenge around kids and food. This book would make a great gift for new parents and is a must-read for parents of older children as well."

—STEPHANIE S. SMITH, PSYD, psychologist, writer at www.drstephaniesmith.com, and advisory board member for www.produceforkids.com

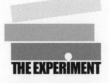

THE EXPERIMENT

BECAUSE EVERY BOOK IS A TEST OF NEW IDEAS

"The unique perspectives of both authors—a physician dedicated to pediatric eating habits and a speech-language pathologist specializing in safe feeding and swallowing—fill this book with multidimensional, helpful information for getting children to eat more healthily and safely. After reading this book you will sharpen your skills in parenting mindfully, feeding confidently, and avoiding picky eating! This book is also ideal for speech-language pathology and occupational therapy students hoping to one day become feeding specialists."

—Dawn Winkelmann, MS, CCC-SLP, speech-language
pathologist and feeding specialist

"This is hands-down the best book available on how to help kids become courageous eaters. Melanie Potock and Dr. Nimali Fernando provide a clear, practical, easy-to-follow road map to guide parents through this often bumpy developmental journey, including the best ways to position an infant for feeding, transition to solid foods, get rid of the pacifier and thumb sucking, and get kids to try new foods, even those with extremely limited food repertoires."

—Lindsey Biel, MA, OTR/L, pediatric occupational therapist,
author of *Sensory Processing Challenges: Effective Clinical Work
with Kids & Teens,* and coauthor of *Raising a Sensory Smart
Child: The Definitive Guide to Helping Your Child with Sensory
Processing Issues*

"Finally, a book that takes on the real root causes of picky eating. Best not to wait for picky eating to begin and read this book now, but if you already have terror at the table help is on its way."

—Kelly Dorfman, MS, LND,
author of *Cure Your Child with Food*

"Dr. Nimali Fernando and Melanie Potock help parents to understand the physical and developmental aspects of learning to eat, including gross motor and fine motor milestones, and how these set the foundation for optimal eating. With a myriad of strategies to help kids explore and learn about food, parents now have an arsenal of healthy interventions from which to draw upon as their child grows."

—Jill Castle, MS, RDN, childhood nutrition expert and
author of *Fearless Feeding*

"Dr. Nimali Fernando and Melanie Potock explain development using real-life examples and provide parents with loads of practical advice for every childhood age and stage. The book is parent- and reader-friendly, while providing a balance of developmental and behavioral information. It also considers the whole child as well as the parent-child partnership needed for healthy feeding, eating, drinking, and nutrition."

—DIANE BAHR, CCC-SLP, CIMI, author of *Nobody Ever Told Me (or My Mother) That! Everything from Bottles and Breathing to Healthy Speech Development*

"Rare is the book that both informs and delightfully entertains and *Raising a Healthy, Happy Eater* does just that. After just a few sentences, I felt like I was sitting at a table with the smartest and most insightful girlfriends—as coauthors Dr. Nimali Fernando and Melanie Potock guided me through each stage of eating throughout a child's life."

—AMANDA MASCIA, founder of The Good Food Factory

"I love the way Dr. Nimali Fernando and Melanie Potock have approached feeding—it's a perfect combination of education and encouragement, which is exactly what parents need to create positive feeding experiences. *Raising a Healthy, Happy Eater* will give parents the tools to approach feeding with confidence—because what could be better than getting feeding advice from a pediatrician and a feeding expert!"

—KIA ROBERTSON, founder of the Eat A Rainbow Project

"Parents want easy solutions, fun strategies, and creative guidance, backed by professional knowledge and mixed with a dose of reality. You'll find the perfect mix with Dr. Nimali Fernando and Melanie Potock—and become well on your way to raising healthy, happy eaters."

—KELLY LESTER, CEO, EasyLunchboxes

ALSO BY MELANIE POTOCK

*Adventures in Veggieland: Help Your Kids Learn to Love
Vegetables with 100 Easy Activities and Recipes*

*Happy Mealtimes with Happy Kids: How to Teach Your Child
About the Joy of Food!*

RAISING A HEALTHY, HAPPY EATER

A PARENT'S HANDBOOK

A Stage-by-Stage Guide to
Setting Your Child on the Path
to Adventurous Eating

NIMALI FERNANDO, MD, MPH
MELANIE POTOCK, MA, CCC-SLP
Foreword by Roshini Raj, MD

THE EXPERIMENT
NEW YORK

The Experiment, LLC
220 East 23rd Street, Suite 600
New York, NY 10010-4658
theexperimentpublishing.com

This book contains the opinions and ideas of its author. It is intended to provide helpful and informative material on the subjects addressed in the book. It is sold with the understanding that the author and publisher are not engaged in rendering medical, health, or any other kind of personal professional services in the book. The author and publisher specifically disclaim all responsibility for any liability, loss, or risk—personal or otherwise—that is incurred as a consequence, directly or indirectly, of the use and application of any of the contents of this book.

The Experiment's books are available at special discounts when purchased in bulk for premiums and sales promotions as well as for fund-raising or educational use. For details, contact us at info@theexperimentpublishing.com.

Library of Congress Cataloging-in-Publication Data
Fernando, Nimali.
  Raising a healthy, happy eater : a parent's handbook-- a stage-by-stage guide to setting your child on the path to adventurous eating / Nimali Fernando, MD, Melanie Potock, CCC-SLP.
    pages cm
  Includes bibliographical references and index.
  1. Children--Nutrition. 2. Children--Health and hygiene. 3. Parent and child. I. Potock, Melanie. II. Title.
  RJ206.F47 2015
  618.92--dc23
                2015003945
ISBN 978-1-61519-268-7
Ebook ISBN 978-1-61519-269-4

Cover design by Laywan Kwan
Cover photograph by Sarah Smith
Author photograph by Daryle Darden
Text design by Pauline Neuwirth, Neuwirth & Associates, Inc.

Manufactured in the United States of America

First printing October 2015
10 9 8 7 6 5

To my devoted husband Daryle and my beautiful, adventurous sons Zane and Asa, who always stand by me and inspire me to live out my dreams. And to my parents who have always been the most kindhearted and enthusiastic supporters of Doctor Yum's mission.

—DR. YUM

There are three people in this world who love me to the moon and back and inspire, support, and guide me every single step of the way: my husband Bob and my two daughters, Mallory and Carly. They make every day a joy—and every family dinner one filled with gratitude. This book is dedicated to them for encouraging me to listen to my heart above all other voices.

—COACH MEL

Contents

FOREWORD
by Roshini Raj, MD

....

The moment your first child is born, you embark on the most rewarding and challenging job you will ever have. At least that's how I felt seven years ago, when I was handed my yowling bundle of joy in the hospital room. I experienced overwhelming love, but I also understood the tremendous responsibility I had for keeping this tiny being safe, healthy, and happy.

As a physician and a medical reporter, the healthy part was (and still is) foremost in my mind, and I vowed to do everything in my power to ensure the good, lasting health of my child. In my field of gastroenterology, I regularly see firsthand the effects of poor nutrition on adult health, and by now we've all heard how our society's poor eating habits have led to epidemics of obesity, diabetes, and even cancer.

The reality is these poor habits start early and are ingrained during childhood, which is why *Raising a Healthy, Happy Eater* is such a vital resource for parents who want to raise healthy children. Drawing on their distinct and vast professional experiences, Coach Mel and Dr. Yum use their expertise to help parents navigate the difficult and often anxiety-provoking world of feeding children. Rather than the usual frustration that parents and children both experience during these food battles, the authors' "joyful" approach to the challenge reminds us that mealtimes are meant to be (and truly can be!) a fun experience for the whole family.

The parenting skills they teach are useful tools for all aspects of parenting, not just for food-related issues. Feeding issues can crop up at any age, so whether you have an infant or a school-age child, this book will help you work with your child in a constructive manner to ensure happy and healthy mealtimes. The book also offers insight into how our sensory systems interact with food and why certain foods may be challenging for little ones—it's this ability to understand what your child is experiencing, rather than just viewing them as being stubborn, that helps frame the food issue as a collaborative rather than combative approach.

Ultimately, you'll begin looking forward to meals with your children, knowing that you're not only sharing love and conversation, but also that you're laying the foundation for good health for the rest of their future.

—ROSHINI RAJ, MD, attending physician at
NYU Langone Medical Center/Tisch Hospital,
Associate Professor of Medicine at
NYU School of Medicine,
and *Today* show contributor

INTRODUCTION
Our Chicken Nugget World: Reality Bites

This book is neither a critique of comfort food nor a condemnation of fast food. Our tone is one of compassion and camaraderie. We all share this world, and it's a world where Dr. Yum's pediatrics office is flanked by a pair of fast-food restaurants, and where Coach Mel taught her children to drink from a straw at one of America's most popular hamburger chains. While there are plenty of healthy "kid food" alternatives discussed in this book, the reality is that we authors—and our own families—have enjoyed a few chicken nuggets from time to time, with extra sweet-and-sour sauce to boot. Frankly, it's a part of the American culture to devour a hot dog at the ballpark or "buttered" popcorn at the movies. Healthy? No. Delicious? Of course!

But for many of our kids today, eating like this isn't the occasional treat. They're bombarded with unhealthy foods from a very early age, thanks to a society that has become focused on convenience, constant snacking, and meals on the run. Most of the food in our world is processed for longer shelf life, and sacrifices nutrition for taste. And if you have a child who falls anywhere on the spectrum of "picky eating," America's food culture reinforces this "tasty treat" eating pattern. In our fast-paced lives, it's easy to allow our children to overindulge or rely on unhealthy options, because we know they'll enjoy them and, importantly, actually eat them. Even if you are the parent who has already started your child on the path to healthy eating, it may only be a matter of time before your kids are faced with the actuality of a junk-food culture. Reality bites: It's a chicken-nugget world out there, and it's unlikely to change overnight.

If you're interested in exploring how to raise adventurous eaters, then this book is for you. We'll walk you through the developmental process of how children learn to eat food of all kinds over time. We'll help you expand your child's diet. We'll show how to use parenting strategies that work both in and out of the kitchen. So, let's bring back family dinners. Let's learn to identify feeding problems before our kids fall into the picky eater trap. Let's pay attention to what we can do as parents to make a difference for our kids, nutritionally, physically, and emotionally. Together, we can create a new world that's a more balanced place to live. Let's create a culture of wellness—for our kids and for our communities. That's why we're here: to guide you on the path to raising healthy, happy eaters.

HOW TO USE THIS BOOK

Keep an eye out for these symbols throughout the book, which will help guide you as you travel on your journey to healthier, joyful mealtimes with your entire family.

 Nimali Fernando, MD, aka Dr. Yum, is the leader of the trek! She's a pediatrician who loves to teach how fresh, real food is essential for a child's health and well-being. Dr. Yum will help guide you with tips about child development, children's nutrition, how to introduce new foods, and how to have lots of fun along the way! She'll be including stories from her own experience working with parents who want to raise adventurous eaters. In fact, she's got a chef's kitchen right in her pediatric office in Virginia! She's your "pediatrician in the kitchen"!

 Melanie Potock, aka Coach Mel, is Dr. Yum's fearless associate who understands how to encourage the more hesitant eaters in your family to participate in food exploration. In real life, Coach Mel is an experienced kids' food coach and a certified speech-language pathologist who specializes in working with selective and picky eaters.

 Seven different "passport stamps" alert you to unique parenting concepts that can be used in the kitchen to raise an adventurous eater. You might be surprised when these parenting mantras spill over into other areas of your life, helping you to raise a brave, joyful, and compassionate child, too!

 The magnifying glass offers "A Closer Look" at any topic, pointing you toward more focused information if you wish to explore a particular topic in greater detail. You can skip it or read it later—it's up to you!

A globe illustrates the "What Kids Eat Around the World" sections, where we explore the wonderful varieties of food that kids from different countries eat and encourage you to expose your children to some exciting and diverse food. We even include unique recipes from various cultures for you to make with your kids! It's fun to look beyond the typical Western palate and offer food with a range of flavors and nutrient profiles. Just like traveling, learning to be an adventurous eater means experiencing new things!

1

THE START OF YOUR CHILD'S FOOD JOURNEY
Parenting the Whole Child

....

Helping families feed their children is more than our daily work: It's our daily love. To see a child pick up the broccoli they "hate" and finally put it in their mouth and smile is what makes us tick. We are Dr. Nimali Fernando (known as Dr. Yum) and Melanie Potock (Coach Mel)—two moms who happen to have careers that focus on family mealtimes. Dr. Yum is a pediatrician who teaches her patients' families how to prepare a healthy diet and thereby prevent illness. Coach Mel is a certified speech-language pathologist with a unique specialty—she's a food coach. Most importantly, we are parents like you, who are invested in raising healthy eaters despite living in a chicken nugget world.

> "What am I making for supper? Why, sweetie, I'm making whatever the hell I want, served with a side of 'eat it or starve.'"
>
> —ANNE TAINTOR, INC.

MELANIE: That's the way I was raised: liver and onions, potato-chip-tuna casserole straight out of *Woman's Day,* and Jell-O ambrosia as a special treat. "Eat it or starve." We had never heard of food allergies, giving up gluten, or (God forbid) not drinking four glasses of milk daily. My relationship with my mom and dad centered on nightly family dinners, served sharply at 1800 military time (that's 6:00 p.m. for you civilians), which started with a prayer and ended with me doing the dishes.

NIMALI: For me, growing up in a Sri Lankan American family, home-cooked meals were a tradition. My mother adapted her cooking to American styles as we grew up—she rotated meals of meat loaf and potatoes between rice and curry dishes—but there was *always* a home-cooked dinner on the table. As a child, helping my mom and siblings prepare food gave me a great foundation of basic cooking skills, as well as an appreciation for how precious time in the kitchen with family can be.

For many families today, the scenario looks rather different. According to a study out of UCLA, working parents are relying on convenience foods and acting as short-order cooks to appease picky appetites at home. Parents don't want to disappoint anyone when it comes to mealtimes, especially their kids. The parent-child relationship is often based on keeping conflict to a minimum. While many American families still eat dinner together, CBS researchers discovered that they do so in the company of the TV and/or while texting or e-mailing on their personal gadgets.[1] Parents and their children are more disconnected. Today's family mealtimes occur less frequently, with fewer opportunities for emotional connections and family bonding, and with more occasions to be distracted by technology.

Times have also changed when it comes to children's health. With the decline in home-cooked meals, increased reliance on convenience foods including packaged foods and fast food, and decreased physical activity, it's no surprise that childhood obesity rates are higher than ever. Approximately 30 percent of American children can be categorized as overweight or obese by body mass index (BMI) standards. Unfortunately, obesity is just the tip of the iceberg. Many children suffer from other diet-related illnesses, despite a normal BMI. Symptoms like poor concentration, lack of energy, gastroesophageal reflux, and chronic constipation may be linked to a poor diet. These problems can then lead to a list of other issues.

Consider a school-aged child who eats a fiber-less diet of the usual "kid-friendly" food such as pepperoni pizza and hamburgers. This diet may lead to chronic constipation, which can lead to bedwetting and urinary tract infections. A child who continues to wet the bed after a certain age could begin to suffer from poor self-esteem and anxiety. An anxiety medication may seem like the answer to this problem, but better nutrition can resolve all of the symptoms. As a pediatrician, Dr. Yum sees scenarios like this every day. If we just connect the dots, so many medical issues can be traced back to diet.

A rise in childhood feeding disorders is also contributing to our nation's nutrition crisis. At least 25 percent of typically developing children are diagnosed with a feeding disorder,[2] defined as the inability to eat a sufficient variety of foods in order to maintain a healthy nutritional status.[3] Feeding disorders are distinct from eating disorders, which center on body image. Feeding disorders encompass the act of feeding a child and the child's willingness to participate. Many consider the "picky eating epidemic" to be a result of the dramatic rise in food allergies and intolerances. Other contributing factors may include sensory integration challenges; the increases in premature births and autism; the evolution of the two-income family and subsequent changes in family lifestyles; or misguided parenting, plain and simple.

The truth is: *Parents want answers.* As we have found in our practices, they're asking for tools to "parent in the kitchen." They want to know how to bring back family dinnertime, how to connect with their children over delicious, healthy food, and how to encourage their most hesitant children to become adventurous eaters.

Feeding your child is an activity packed with emotions: It's about nurturing, loving, and being a responsible parent. Food *is* love, in so many ways. But when your child has eating difficulties, life takes an unexpected turn, and mealtimes become the most stressful periods of the day. Feeding troubles may begin with breast-feeding challenges, during the transition to solid foods, or maybe even later down the road. At some point, "picky eater" may become a common term in your family's vocabulary. And let's face it: Whether your child's an adventurous eater or a hesitant one, we're living in a chicken nugget world. Fast food and the same old kids' menus appear at every corner, and parents fall right into the "kid food" trap—a mire of macaroni and cheese, French fries, and burgers. Exasperated parents are quick to rely on the one strategy that they know will work: "Just give him some nuggets—he'll always eat those!" Before long, vegetables and other nutritious foods simply don't appear on the child's plate any more. After all, parents wonder, why be wasteful? The kid won't eat them anyway.

Having a child who doesn't eat like his peers or another sibling can be maddening. As one mother told Coach Mel, "When you have a picky eater, you have so many opportunities to fail as a parent . . . starting with breakfast, lunch, and dinner." Why will one child eat anything and everything, yet for another, the world comes to an end if you put green beans on his plate? The answer to that question is complicated, but *Raising a Healthy, Happy Eater* will break it down, step-by-step, so that you consider all the factors that impact your child as they build their eating skills. Learning to suck, bite, chew, and swallow a variety of foods easily, with interest and enthusiasm, is part of child development. But it's really about parenting, too—and if you've taken the time to open this book, pat yourself on the back. *You* have taken an important step in ensuring that your parenting skills attend to every aspect of your child's life—including mealtimes.

Having a consistent approach to mealtimes can help avoid so many of the feeding issues children encounter. The techniques you'll find in this book may be different from what you're used to. One's parenting style usually comes from a mix of life experience, family background, culture, and the community around us. To learn to parent differently than what you've been shown for years takes effort and practice, and can feel strange at first. However, shifting your parenting style, especially during mealtimes, can spill over into other aspects of family life in a very positive way. When mealtime experiences are more pleasant, time away from the table becomes more pleasant, too. The opposite is true as well—when family life is running smoothly, mealtimes tend to be a happy time for everyone.

Let's take the example of limit testing. Around the ages of three to five, children can constantly and deliberately test limits, trying to map the boundaries of appropriate behaviors. Themes like, "If I cry and scream, will I get what I want?" or "How many times do I have to ask for this toy before Mommy will change her mind?" frequently run through a preschooler's head. Understanding this stage of development, we realize that being consistent and setting boundaries are key to helping a child map out those limits in the most efficient way.

This approach is just as applicable to other aspects of life. When a child is having a hard time going to preschool, seasoned teachers know that a quick morning drop-off makes for the easiest transition, despite the initial tears it may cause. If parents linger at the door or spend time in the classroom with the child to try to make it easier, the transition can become confusing and prolong the child's adjustment. In the same way, having clear, consistent rules about eating can help kids adjust to new foods. On the contrary, not setting rules and limits at this age may create a resistance to new foods, further prolonging your child's path to a healthy diet.

Whether parenting in the kitchen or outside of it, don't forget to have fun! Joy is so essential when interacting with children. Too often as parents, we can get stuck feeling like all our decisions are incredibly important, and that if we make a mistake we won't have an opportunity to fix it. For many parents, this pressure can take the joy out of parenting. But a positive attitude is essential, and in our experience it's the main ingredient to raising an adventurous eater—it's the secret sauce, so to speak! You will notice that fun comes up in different ways throughout the book. Taking the time to giggle at the sound of the broccoli squeaking makes for a happier, more willing broccoli eater. As you enjoy your child's journey toward adventurous eating, you may find that child blossoming into a junior foodie! While that journey does not always happen quickly, enjoy all of the accomplishments and experiences of today.

As feeding professionals, we see a wide range of children, each one with his or her distinct eating preferences and food journeys. This is true even within our own families. We each have two children vastly different from one another in many ways, including their journeys with food. Parents tend to have initial expectations about how their child will learn to eat, and if it is their second child, those expectations may be heavily influenced by the experiences with their first. Sometimes it creates pressure and parents blame themselves when children don't progress in the way that they had imagined. It's easy to wonder why your child isn't eating, learning, or speaking as well as an older sibling or a friend's kid. But remember that every child is different, and there is joy to be found in each step of a child's journey. If your first child was a relatively adventurous eater and didn't go through any picky phases, you may be surprised if your second child refuses many foods. Just know that you can still enjoy the baby steps it sometimes takes to help that child along, and that no two children will ever be exactly the same.

Parenting the whole child, "body, brain, and soul," is a concept vital to our philosophy. Learning to be an adventurous eater involves the entire body, including gross motor skills, fine motor skills, and cognitive development—*plus* an emotional component. As parents, you have the honor of serving as your child's guide on this spectacular journey! We'll share information about how your baby, toddler, or young child's development directly influences the type of eater she'll be and, more importantly, how you can support her to be the best eater she can be at each stage. From food choices during pregnancy to your child's first bites of solid food, from preparing dinners to spending mealtimes with your child, we hope to help you make the kitchen and the wonderful food that comes out of it the heart of your family.

Your Parenting Passport

Throughout this book you'll find seven parenting strategies to keep in mind so that you and your child both thrive on the road to adventurous eating. By following these guides, you'll nourish your child not just nutritionally, but emotionally, too. In essence, these strategies comprise your Parenting Passport, represented by passport stamps that remind you of the right direction to take. These stamps serve as prompts to help you navigate challenges along the way.

 Celebrate each step in this journey—like any adventure, the more fun you bring to the experience, the better! Remember, family mealtimes are about the *family* experience more than the meal itself. We'll walk you through the steps your child can take to become a lifelong adventurous eater.

 Understanding your child's developmental stage allows you to put yourself in his shoes, enabling you to parent both respectfully *and* effectively. In many parenting challenges, a respectful and caring approach can guide the child while sustaining his unique spirit. Mealtimes are the perfect opportunity to adopt this philosophy.

 With any new experience, it's natural to feel a bit scared, especially if this is your first child. But we never want fear to be a roadblock to moving forward. Armed with the knowledge of how children learn to eat, you'll feel brave, plus you'll learn to expect the natural ebb and flow of feeding.

 Waiting is a "magic" parenting technique. Although you are your child's guide, your role is to show her the way—not pull her along. We'll give you tips on how to patiently observe your child and allow her to find her way, while boosting the motor skills directly related to eating.

Understanding what comes next in your child's development is the key to proactive parenting. Like any other road trip, it's a good idea to know what's around the corner! And how you react to what you encounter is up to you. By anticipating the next steps during mealtime experiences, you can set your child up for success.

Your child will thrive on knowing specific boundaries and will respond to your gentle, consistent guidance throughout his life. Consistency is crucial for building new skills and habits effectively, especially when you're gathered around the family table.

Be present. Observe your child's unique needs during different developmental stages. Mindfulness also applies to the behaviors we model around our children, setting the stage for successful eating.

• •

We hope that the upcoming chapters bring insight into how to raise a healthy, happy eater while you and your child explore exciting and delicious foods. Even if you find yourself in some challenging food situations, know that there's often a silver lining to be found and ways to bring out the best in your kids. We also hope the underlying lessons of these chapters will be helpful when it comes to other aspects of parenting. So get ready, buckle up, and enjoy the adventure!

SIGHTS, SOUNDS, AND EXPLORATION
Understanding the Sensory System

Can you name a food that gives you the "heebie-jeebies"? It may not be accurate medical terminology, but just the thought of the heebie-jeebies evokes a shudder and a wince, stirring up a memory of a certain texture or taste that you recall as "repulsive." Your sensory system, which includes seven different neural pathways, may have already communicated to your brain that you are *never* going to try a raw oyster . . . or calf brains . . . or . . . green beans.

Yes, green beans. For young children who are slowly experiencing the world, including new foods, green beans may cause alarm bells to sound until their sensory system adapts to the sight, smell, touch, taste, and even the sound of green beans as they *smoosh* between their teeth. Older children who don't have repeated exposure to a new food may experience the same alarm bells when the traditional green bean casserole appears at Thanksgiving dinner. For some, the reaction may be a simple turned-up nose, but for children who have difficulties with sensory integration, it might include gagging, extreme protesting, or a reaction that appears to be out of proportion to something we consider simple: just trying a green bean.

More than fifty years ago, Dr. Jean Ayres, an occupational therapist and outstanding researcher, introduced the theory of sensory integration: the study of how the brain processes information from the entire sensory system. Lots of sensory input constantly flows into the brain to be organized. For example, consider how a simple change in our environment floods the brain with sensations as we step outside into our backyards on a sunny day: bright light, outdoor aromas, heat on our skin, birds chirping, and dogs barking. Even our movement through space is registered, compared to past experiences, and then organized so that we may react appropriately. Our brain then begins to ask itself, "Which signal is important? Which input can be discarded at this time? Which information applies to what I'm doing at this very moment?" Making each decision efficiently requires a well-coordinated brain, and the entire process is nothing short of amazing.[4]

"Sensory integration puts it all together," writes Dr. Jean Ayres in *Sensory Integration and the Child.* "Imagine peeling and eating an orange. You sense the orange through your eyes, nose, mouth, the skin on your hands and fingers, and also the muscles and joints inside your fingers, hand, arms and mouth. . . . All the sensations from your hands and fingers somehow come together in one place in your brain," which allows you to make decisions on how to peel and eat the orange.[5]

Coach Mel's Tip:
Your Sensory System Is Your Body's GPS
Think of your body's sensory system like your own personal GPS, guiding your internal self through the external world. All parts of the system need to be organized and communicate with each other, sending the proper signals to guide you accurately throughout your day. If one system isn't functioning well, it will impact how well the other systems operate, and you might struggle on your journey.

Infants are exposed to brand-new sensations every single day. It takes time for babies' sensory systems to adapt to the ever-changing input they receive from the world. They may be unable to ignore certain stimuli that wouldn't bother an adult or under-react to some stimuli if their sensory systems are less organized. And the premature infant, who enters the world with an immature nervous system, will be less adaptable than a full-term baby.

For example, as you're reading this book, you may be relaxing on your front porch. Sounds are all around you: A car drives by your house; neighbors are chatting in the yard across the street; birds are chirping. A slight breeze drifts across your face, shifting a strand of hair that tickles your cheek. The new shoes you chose to wear today are a bit tight and the scent of that new sunscreen you applied earlier is strong in the heat. The iced tea you're sipping is getting warm and condensation on the glass is getting your hand a little wet. But does any of that stop you from processing the information you're reading? Probably not, because you've experienced those sensations before and your brain tells you, "Just ignore it—keep reading." But if you're someone with a sensory processing disorder, you may have trouble taking in all this information bombarding your senses, causing you to react in an atypical way.

Simultaneously, your brain will be attempting to pull up prior information and memories, so that it can compare the current sensory input to previously stored "data," thus helping you decide how to respond to the tickle on your cheek, or the neighbors chatting in the background, or the most important task, processing what you're reading. This happens because your sensory system has become more organized over time and you've learned to integrate certain stimuli while reacting in a meaningful way to others.

Learning to enjoy new foods also requires a balanced sensory processing system. An overactive system (e.g., a child screaming at the feel of a squishy banana in her hands), or an underactive system (e.g., swallowing bites of food whole because of poor awareness of exactly where that food is in the mouth), can hinder developmental progress in learning to eat. The less exposure you have to a variety of textures, tastes, and temperatures, the fewer opportunities you have to store relevant information in your brain for later comparison. If you've never eaten carrot puree or green bean casserole, and you've had little to no experience with anything similar to those foods, there are hardly any memories for you to retrieve and expand on. Plus, if your sensory system isn't working properly, you may feel so overwhelmed by the various inputs that the brain's retrieval process can't operate efficiently, and you begin to have a meltdown. It's all just too much.

THE SEVEN SENSES

Speaking of processing . . . do you remember reading on page 13 that there are seven pathways for information to be processed and stored via our sensory system? Something doesn't quite add up here—aren't there *five* senses? Most of us learned to name them in elementary school: sight, sound, smell, taste, and touch. We'll let you in on a secret. There are two more: the vestibular sense, or balance, and the sense of proprioception—awareness of your body position. Both pathways contribute to how a child explores new foods. As we walk through all seven senses and how they relate to feeding, we'll approach it from toddlerhood, when a child's sensory system has had a few years to gather information, store it in the brain, and begin to retrieve it as she explores a variety of foods:

1. The Vestibular System—Balance: Every parent knows the importance of a balanced diet, but what does the sense of balance have to do with trying new foods? Our sense of balance and movement, originating in the inner ear and known as the vestibular system, is the foundation for all fine motor skills. When your child picks up her first roly-poly pea with her tiny thumb and forefinger, that's demonstrating some very "fine" fine motor skills! But did you know that biting, chewing, and swallowing are also fine motor skills, and that a child requires adequate balance and stability to perform those skills with ease?

If you were presented with a new food, one that you were not sure of, would you be patient enough to try it? Not if most of your energy is devoted to keeping your balance and moving a fork through space so that you don't stab yourself. It's exhausting! As a feeding specialist, Coach Mel frequently sees this scenario when visiting households. Young children are seated in square, plastic booster seats with their feet dangling. As they wobble at the table, they often have one hand gripping the table edge or the booster seat tray in order to remain steady. Little toes are often braced under the tray or reaching for any object to prop themselves against so that tiny hands can remain steady and snag a piece of food. Children may fatigue quickly before finishing a meal.

In chapter 4, we'll provide specific tips on how to correctly position your children in a high chair so that the vestibular system and the corresponding muscles that support the trunk don't have to work quite so hard.

Thank goodness for our vestibular system! Without it, kids would never learn to pick up a piece of corn on the cob and nibble from one end to another. They would never learn to hold an ice cream cone upright and gauge their movement so that vanilla soft-serve ends up on the tongue, and not up the nose!

Coach Mel's Tip: Try Sitting Like a Toddler

To get a sense of what it can be like for a toddler to balance at mealtime, try this: Sit on a bar stool at the local diner and order a piece of pie (or other dish that you can eat one-handed). Dangle your feet—absolutely do *not* rest them on the footrest. Keep one hand floating in the air to maintain your balance, but do not touch the counter. Now, pick up your fork with the other hand and eat the pie. Feel your abs tighten to hold your trunk in place? Can you feel your shoulders tense to stabilize your arm and hand as they move through space? How well can you cut, stab, and lift the piece of pie on your fork without spilling any on your lap? For a toddler's growing body—one with less muscle control—this is extraordinarily difficult.

Getting tired yet? Your vestibular system and your muscles are hard at work as you float in space and try to eat that pie, but you're not an astronaut. Phew! That's hard work!

2. The Proprioceptive System—Body Awareness: Ever wonder why some people are such naturals on the dance floor and others have two left feet? If motor coordination is not your forte, you can blame some of it on your poor sense of proprioception.

Proprioception refers to our own awareness of where our various body parts are in space, and how much strength, effort, and coordination must be utilized to move each part effectively. Proprioception can affect not only your ability on the dance floor, but also your ability to eat a salad. Without a solid sense of where your hand is you're likely to stick the fork in your cheek!

We've all done it: When you tip a tall iced tea glass toward your mouth much too quickly and end up with ice cascading down your shirt, blame it on inferior proprioceptive skills. Toddlers are developing their sense of proprioception as they practice motor skills, such as feeding themselves with a spoon or using a fork to stab a cooked baby carrot. Push too hard and the carrot breaks into pieces; hold the fork at the wrong angle and the carrot becomes orange mush. As a child's muscles contract and stretch with each attempt at piercing the carrot, the brain receives proprioceptive input and communicates how to adjust the movement in order to get the carrot onto the fork tines. With practice, eventually a child learns to stab the carrot and to fine-tune the movements so that the carrot ends up in her mouth at last! In chapter 4, we'll walk you through gross and fine motor development and offer strategies for guiding your child as new experiences hone his sense of proprioception.

3. The Visual System—Sight: Every great chef tells us that we first "feast with our eyes." Within the first few days of life, newborn babies utilize the sense of sight by gazing into a mother's eyes. Sight is often the first sense that children use when considering how to interact with a new food. As babies develop and become toddlers, sight becomes even more important at mealtimes. Raw broccoli isn't steamed broccoli and definitely isn't broccoli casserole! Toddlers prefer foods that are easily identified, and casseroles are not easily identified.

4. The Tactile System—Touch: The skin is rich in nerve endings, especially on the palm of the hands and the fingers. But the inside of the mouth may have even more! Babies are programmed to explore the world with the hands and mouth. One of the first fine motor skills that an infant acquires is the ability to bring their hands, and eventually, a toy, to their open mouths. This innate drive to explore the world via hands, fingers, and mouth is also the first step to learning about new foods. In chapter 4, we'll discuss "baby-led weaning," a feeding model that emphasizes a child's need to learn about new foods by grasping, squeezing, and squishing them until eventually, the food makes its way into the child's mouth.

5. The Auditory System—Hearing: Did you know that each food has a unique sound? The sense of hearing involves more than just the whir of a blender or the chop, chop, chop on a cutting board as sound waves bounce against the eardrum. We also hear ourselves crunch a cracker through bone conduction, where the sound waves travel through the bones in our skulls to our inner ear. And sound is a larger component of our eating experience than many of us realize.

What's sound got to do with eating, or more specifically, with taste? Discovering how the sound of a crunching potato chip affects flavor is more than just curiosity.[6] Professor Charles Spence, who leads University of Oxford's Crossmodal Research Laboratory, studied how the sound that food makes in our mouths influences our perception of freshness. Why is it that some kids prefer a vegetable that snaps and crunches rather than one that is boiled? We're not sure, but the sensations that kids experience in their mouths creates memories that later influence their preferences.

Background sounds in the environment may also influence taste. Spence conducted an experiment in which individuals were given four identical pieces of toffee. The subjects ate two toffee pieces while listening to the low pitch of brass instruments. Two other pieces were eaten while listening to the higher pitch of a piano. The subjects rated the pieces eaten during the piano music as "sweet," and the pieces eaten during the lower pitched music "bitter."[7]

Perhaps future research might apply Spence's work to children learning to try new foods. Would certain tones be more soothing while eating? Would certain music in the school cafeteria help children eat faster or even choose more nutritious foods? "A feast for the eyes" may one day turn out to be "a feast for the eyes and ears" as we consider all the possibilities.[8]

Coach Mel's Tip:
Create Music in Your Mouth

When we crunch on a carrot, the sound waves not only travel through the air and into our ears, stimulating the eardrum, but also travel via the bones in our face and skull! Kids can experience the sensation of bone conduction by plugging their ears with their fingers as they chew. Does the crunch sound louder? What happens to the sound when you chew with an open mouth versus a closed mouth? Try different foods—you might be surprised at the difference in the crunch of a carrot, jicama, and celery. It's music in your mouth!

6. Olfactory System—Smell: Research demonstrates that our sense of smell is closely linked to our emotions and memory.[9] But it doesn't take a scientist to explain that the aroma of freshly baked cookies reminds some of us of cooking with Grandma (and how much we loved her), or that the smell of roasted turkey conjures up Thanksgiving and all the emotions that go along with the holiday. Even tiny babies learn that the smell of their mother's breast milk means they are about to be fed and the sweet scent helps them identify their mom.[10] If you could peer into the human brain, the physical link between smell, emotion, and memory would be clear to see. The olfactory nerve is near the amygdala, the emotional center of the brain, and the hippocampus, the brain's memory center. For young children exploring new foods, just one unpleasant olfactory experience—the sulfur-like smell of rotten hard-boiled egg, for example—can influence future interactions with that same food. But how does smell influence taste when the food has already entered the mouth?

First, picture the inside of your nose, where there are millions of receptor cells that detect odors. Next, picture your tongue, where receptor cells for flavor (taste buds) detect five different tastes. Now, imagine breathing. It is air that carries aromas to the receptor cells and then to the olfactory nerve and the brain. If the air is circulating in your mouth while you chew and you're not suffering from a stuffy nose, the olfactory nerve will be stimulated while you're eating. Plug your nose—and you essentially stop your sense of taste.

Coach Mel's Tip: Eat a Jelly Bean

Try this with your kids! Here's a fun experiment, described in *Scientific American* online, demonstrating how we need to smell food in order to truly experience its flavor. For children over age three, blindfold your kids and give them a jelly bean to chew with their mouths closed for a few seconds, *while they plug their nose*. While they will be able to sense sweet or sour, they may not be able to identify the exact flavor. The odor molecules can't reach the olfactory nerve without airflow. Quick, unplug that nose and open your mouth so that the olfactory nerve can do its thing! Ah, now you can taste it! What flavor was it?[11]

7. The Gustatory System—Taste: The sense of taste is not only enhanced by the sense of smell, but also by thousands of nerve endings that detect unique properties of food. For example, some receptors detect the coolness of mint or the warmth of a spice, like chili powder. Combine those sensations with the input from thousands of taste buds found on the tongue, roof of the mouth, and throat, and the perception of taste is a fascinating interplay of sensations. Scientists have identified five different tastes: sweet, sour, bitter, salty, and umami. Umami is the savory taste you experience when you taste food like aged cheese or fatty steak seared over an open grill. Proteins break down and reveal L-glutamate, the molecule responsible for the umami taste. It is challenging to describe, but delicious to experience!

When it comes to sensitivity to taste, researchers believe that approximately 25 percent of the population are "super-tasters" who taste more intensely,[12] 25 percent are "non-tasters" on the other end of the spectrum, and the remaining 50 percent are somewhere in the middle. Supertasters may have more than sixteen times the number of papillae (the bumps on the tongue that house the taste buds) than the average tongue, which has approximately 10,000.[13] Dr. Spence, the expert on understanding our perception of taste, notes that recent research by Professor Gary Pickering at Canada's Brock University reveals that supertasters have an extreme olfactory experience, too. It's also possible that supertasters are more sensitive to different textures in their mouths. Could your child be a supertaster? If so, he'll need time to adjust to new food adventures.

The kitchen would be a boring place without our amazing sensory systems allowing our bodies to react with precision timing. Without the senses of smell and taste, eating a delectable meal would be a chore. Without the ability to feel the warmth of freshly baked bread in our hands or hear the squirt of a fresh cherry tomato as it pops between our teeth, how would we experience food? If we were never allowed to see food, would the dining-out experience be as satisfying? What would life be like without our balance and coordination to guide our hands to our mouths and keep our bodies upright as we enjoy a nice slice of pie? How fortunate we are to have a sensory system that operates like a beautiful symphony with each sensation playing its own instrument to help us understand every property of food!

A CLOSER LOOK:
Sensory Processing Disorder

For children with sensory processing challenges, often termed sensory processing disorder (previously called sensory integration disorder), eating can be a challenging experience. The sensations from the sight, smell, taste, and feel of foods may be too intense, causing the child to overreact. Or, the input may not be strong enough, making the child less aware and causing underreaction.

In fact, we *all* have good and not-so-good sensory days. But for children who experience the world of food via a disorganized sensory system, the signs of discomfort can range from extremely selective food choices to the more garden-variety "picky eating." That's because sensory processing disorder (SPD) is a spectrum disorder, ranging from mild to severe. Plus, parenting styles influence how a child experiences food, and in turn, a hesitant eater influences how his parents "parent." Factor in the delicate daily life of a child with SPD, and you may have a perfect storm for developing a feeding disorder. If you're encountering feeding obstacles that appear to be sensory related, talk to your pediatrician or speech-language pathologist (SLP), who will likely refer your child to be evaluated by an occupational therapist (OT). Remember, kids with SPD have a wide range of symptoms that can vary from day to day, depending on how well their sensory systems are operating at that particular time. A pediatric OT who focuses on feeding skills may ask if your child is experiencing any of the following symptoms:

- Shudders, gags, or vomits when attempting to try certain foods
- Avoids specific types of food (e.g., purees or chewy foods)
- Is fearful of trying new foods
- Insists on only eating certain brands of food
- Is unable to eat or does not eat well unless at home
- Limits self to food at a specific temperature
- Prefers bland foods and refuses most savory or intense flavors
- Craves intense flavors

- Over-chews food
- Under-chews food and attempts to swallow large pieces
- Overstuffs mouth
- Requires liquids to swallow most bites of food
- Underreacts to hot and/or spicy foods
- Overreacts or underreacts to odors
- Consistently "slumps" at the table or is unable to stay in seat
- Has difficulty achieving gross or fine motor skill milestones (see page 27), especially those related to eating

These are just a few signs that may indicate your child could benefit from occupational therapy to address sensory processing challenges associated with feeding skills, even if your child is in feeding therapy with another professional, often an SLP. If roadblocks are getting in the way of your child enjoying mealtimes, please chat with your pediatrician. Learning to eat a variety of foods is an adventure, and one that should be pleasant for everyone in the family. For more information on feeding therapy, please refer to chapter 13.

As you embark on your child's feeding journey, keep in mind that each child is unique and will have different perceptions that influence daily experiences. We all have distinct sensory systems that change over time, so your child's sensory GPS may offer different routes than you had planned. Whether you take the straight and steady path or end up on a detour that requires a bit of extra support, we'll provide the roadside tips to help you parent consistently.

PACK YOUR BAGS
AND HERE WE GO!
Birth to Six Months

You may be thinking, "Birth to six months? How much is there to know about breast and bottle feeding?" The answer: too much to tell you in this itsy bitsy chapter! Baby's development in the first six months of life is prepping him for the delicious future of crunchy apples, smooth butternut squash risotto, and crispy kale chips. In fact, the developmental process of feeding starts while your baby is still in the womb. It continues when baby is placed on Mommy's belly for "tummy time" and later as baby begins to bring his hands to his mouth. You might be surprised what early skills are necessary to build a successful foundation for adventurous eating!

Although you may not have started your baby on solid foods yet, there are myriad ways that your baby is experiencing the world that may be influencing his future food choices. It is exciting to know that you can already shape your child's eating habits. Just like talking to babies or playing music for them in the first few months can impact their later speech and cognition, parents can expose children to taste and feeding experiences *long* before they put spoons of pureed veggies in their mouths. Let the road to adventurous eating begin!

The combination of taste and smell allows us to experience flavor. The first taste sensations are experienced in the womb, as a fetus floating in the amniotic fluid. The gustatory, or taste system, develops in a fetus as early as the first trimester, with taste buds (papillae) forming by the tenth week of gestation. These tastes buds begin to function early in the second trimester, and by late gestation, the distribution of papillae appear similar to that of an adult. The olfactory system responsible for smell begins to develop around eight weeks with the olfactory bulb in the brain, and smell receptors start to form. Somewhere between the sixteenth and thirty-sixth week, amniotic fluid is able to flow freely into the fetal nasal passages, and there is evidence of smell sensations at around twenty-eight to twenty-nine weeks.[14]

Flavors can enter the amniotic fluid from a mother tasting them (like sweet or salty food) or inhaling scents (like tobacco smoke or perfumed products). In one study, mothers were randomized to either drink or not drink carrot juice during their last trimester of pregnancy and first three months of breast-feeding. At age six months, those babies whose mothers drank the carrot juice were more likely to accept a carrot-flavored cereal and make fewer distasteful expressions (or "yuck faces") than those whose mothers did not drink the carrot juice.[15] It's amazing to think that we can start modeling healthy eating habits before a baby is born!

That taste experience continues after birth. When mothers nurse their babies, many of the flavors in the food they eat are secreted into the breast milk. Therefore, it appears that breast-feeding can provide a much more varied range of flavors to infants than formula. If you are an expectant mother and are considering breast-feeding, know that this may give your baby a head start toward becoming an adventurous eater. It is not hard to imagine why babies raised in cultures where spicy foods are often consumed seem to have little difficulty adjusting to a spicy diet at an early age. Those babies have been tasting spices since before birth. As you will see throughout the next chapters, children in many cultures throughout the world seem to adjust more easily to complex-tasting foods than in Western cultures. If you're an expectant mother (and manage to emerge from the depths of morning sickness), know that eating a healthy variety of fruits, vegetables, herbs, and spices may be showing your baby how to enjoy a green smoothie with pineapple and ginger in a few short years. Continuing that flavorful diet while breast-feeding may make that journey even easier.

Some mothers may worry that their babies may have an increased risk of food allergies if they consume certain "high-risk" foods like peanuts before birth, and some research has supported that theory. However, the most recent research has shown the opposite. One large study demonstrated that in a group of mothers who are not allergic to peanuts, those who ate the largest dose of peanuts and/or tree nuts had infants who were at the lowest risk of developing a nut allergy.[16]

Certainly, there may be circumstances that may not allow you to breast-feed your child, including health concerns for mother or baby. If breast-feeding is not the path that you and your child travel, know that there are *plenty* of opportunities for the formula-fed baby to encounter exciting tastes, including experiencing new flavors in the prenatal environment and when they first start solid foods at around six months. We hope to provide a foundation of information that will help you make decisions on what is best for you, your child, and your family.

GROSS MOTOR SKILL DEVELOPMENT

- How the whole body's muscle development influences your child's feeding journey
- Parenting Proactively: Why tummy time now leads to happy mealtimes later

Gross motor skills involve the larger parts of the body, including reaching with your arms and kicking with your legs. Crawling, jumping, running, and even rolling over for the very first time are all gross motor skills. Throughout *Raising a Healthy, Happy Eater*, we highlight some of the gross motor skills necessary to develop future feeding skills. A newborn baby placed on her mother's chest is already beginning to develop gross motor skills. Her trunk muscles engage in order to learn to control flailing arms and legs. Over time, baby garners more control, and by age three months, she can hold her beautiful head steady when you raise her up to kiss her forehead. Gross motor development begins with the strength and stabilization of the trunk and over time extends to the hands, feet, and head. By six months, baby's trunk has become strong enough that she is beginning to sit up on her own, although she may require some support for added stability. These next six months are a crucial time for strengthening gross motor skills, so that by six months, baby can sit and begin to explore solid foods. Gross motor skills are the foundation for developing age-appropriate fine motor skills.

 At this very moment, as you're reading this, you're parenting proactively. You're taking the time to learn how gross motor skills directly influence your baby's ability to eat first foods, like the scrumptious roasted sweet potato and banana recipe coming up in the next chapter.

How to Guide Your Child: Gross Motor Skills

In 1994, the Back to Sleep campaign, now called Safe to Sleep, was created in order to educate parents and child care providers about the associated risk of sudden infant death syndrome (SIDS) when placing baby on his belly to sleep. This vital campaign helped save many babies from SIDS, then the leading cause of death in infants. However, mindful of these risks, many parents avoided placing their babies face down in the daytime. Tummy time is not only safe when babies are awake and under supervision, but also important to gross motor development. A lack of infant tummy time can result in a number of issues, including delayed gross motor skills and a flattened head shape (plagiocephaly).

 ### Dr. Yum's Tip: Give Your Baby Tummy Time
Let your baby spend time on his tummy from early on. In the first few weeks after birth, the most natural method is to lay him against your chest. For most babies, the umbilical stump should not get in the way of a comfortable prone position. You may be surprised to see how even in the first days,

your baby may be able to extend his neck and "lift" his head! When you lay baby down for naps, try positioning him on his tummy and see how comfortable he is in that position. Catnaps are a great chance to get tummy time, *but make sure to supervise a baby in this position by keeping your palm lightly on his body.* Be sure to place him face up at night and during daytime naps when he cannot be closely supervised.

Babies have an easier time with digestion when they are resting on the belly. It's also a great way for babies to get a different view of the world. In the prone position, a baby will naturally try to lift his head to follow the sights and sounds around him. These exercising movements will be the first "workouts" that will help him build strength in the neck and back muscles, eventually allowing him to roll over, sit unsupported, and crawl. Since fine motor and oral motor skills are dependent on gross motor skills, exercising muscles during tummy time can help make sure your baby is ready for solid foods at six months.

 Coach Mel's Tip: How to Position Your Baby for Breast- or Bottle-feeding
In her book *Nobody Ever Told Me (or My Mother) That!*, speech-language pathologist Diane Bahr, MS, CCC-SLP explains the best positions for breast- or bottle-feeding. She suggests following these guidelines:

- Keep baby's head, neck, and body in a straight line, careful not to allow the head and neck to extend backward. Bahr explains: "Hyperextension of the head and neck can cause irregular patterns to occur in your baby's mouth. These patterns include wide jaw movement, excessive tongue protrusion, tongue humping and mounding and biting down for stability."[17]

- Position your baby at a forty-five degree angle (or more for older babies) so that her ear is above her mouth. This ensures that fluid does not enter the tiny eustachian tubes, which lead from the back of the throat to behind the eardrum. Fluid accumulation behind the eardrum can lead to infection and hearing loss.

- In addition, Coach Mel recommends swaddling or positioning your full-term baby so that her hands are at midline with elbows bent and on the center of her chest, and her knees are slightly bent. A pillow or the crook of your arm works perfectly to provide this tiny bit of flexion. Bring your baby's hands toward the center of her chest, tucking her elbows into her sides with your arm wrapped around her. You can also give your baby a footrest, like a pillow or even the crook of your elbow with your other arm. Pressing her feet down and bending her knees will help her feel more stable. This gentle support gives her the same feeling of contentment she had *in utero*. Please note that preemies require special positioning, and it's important to follow the guidelines established while your baby was in the nursery, which may be different than described here.

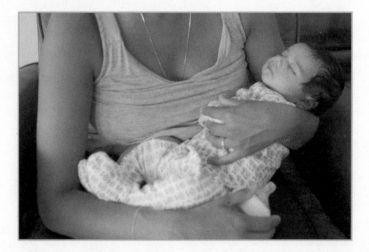

FINE MOTOR SKILL DEVELOPMENT

- Babies learn that fingers move independently from arms and hand
- How early fine motor skills lead to picking up and holding first foods
- Parenting Mindfully: How purposeful play leads to building new skills

All fine motor control stems from the trunk, so tummy time does more than just build strong muscles for sitting up and crawling. You'll also be establishing a base for baby's fine motor skills. These involve the extremities, but with "finer" movement, such as gently waving "bye-bye" for the first time by opening and shutting little fingers, or grasping a soft toy to bring to the mouth for chewing. Wiggling toes in the bathwater is also a fine motor skill. From birth to three months, babies learn to control the gross motor skill of moving their arms through space by bringing their hands to midline. This position allows baby to explore his hands and fingers with his mouth. By three months of age, baby can now grasp a teething toy when you place it in the palm of his hand and then, on his own, bring it to his mouth. Can you picture your baby using that new skill to hold his own bottle with your help?

By six months of age, baby is quite good at banging those same objects and squishing soft toys to make them squeak. He will intentionally release his grip and drop things just so that he can watch them fall. Are you envisioning your baby grabbing pieces of sweet potato or avocado, only to drop them over the edge of the high chair to watch them *splat* on the kitchen floor? These early fine motor skills are the prerequisites to playing with food, one of the most important steps your baby can take in the early stages of this journey.

How to Guide Your Child: Fine Motor Skills

Once baby has begun to adjust to all the sight and sounds of his brand-new world, you can begin to encourage him to put toys in his mouth. Choose soft toys that are easy for his fists to grasp. At first, his arm movements will not be smooth or controlled, but as his shoulders and neck muscles grow stronger with tummy time, he will gain better control over his limbs.

 As you spend time playing with your child on the floor, you're not only enjoying the interaction, you're also being purposeful. You're observing and responding to your child while focusing on the connection you have with him. You're intentionally challenging him just enough—it's the sweet spot that keeps the play fun yet focused on building new skills.

Likewise, as he gains control of his arms, he'll get better control of his hands and fingers. Be sure to give him toys that yield varied textures, shapes, and sounds as he mouths them. Babies are programmed to explore and you're their guide! Once baby is able to lift her shoulders while lying on a play mat, place toys just beyond her reach, so that she learns to reach an inch farther to snag them. Can she grab it when it's directly in front of her or to either side? How about when she is learning to sit up with your help? Can she reach forward and grab the toy on the carpet with one hand, even if you put it on the opposite side? Be sure to exercise each side of her body equally. We don't expect kids to have "hand preferences" until age three, and the more they work each side of their bodies, the more they work each side of the brain!

 Dr. Yum's Tip:
Well Baby Checks Are Important!

Don't forget those well baby checks. Not only do pediatricians check your baby's growth, but they also make sure that your baby has just the right level of muscle tone for his age. With a few physical exam techniques, pediatricians are able to detect if a baby has too much or too little muscle tone, and if he may need more attention in certain gross motor skills and fine motor skills. Well baby checks are a great opportunity for you to make sure his skills are on target, and if they are not, to get suggestions from your pediatrician on helping him progress.

ORAL MOTOR SKILL DEVELOPMENT

- How oral reflexes prepare baby for learning how to eat
- When spitting up becomes a problem
- Parenting Mindfully: Being sensitive to baby's cues of fullness.

Oral motor skills are fine motor skills specific to the oral cavity—i.e., the mouth. A baby's mouth is the center of communication from the moment of birth, when that triumphant cry first erupts! In the first six months, as baby learns to control the jaw, the lips, the tongue, and even the soft palate, she'll begin to communicate intentionally with vowel-like coos and specific cries for "I'm hungry," "I'm tired," and "I'm hurt." Mouth movements for speech and feeding skills are closely related and get their start via infant reflexes.

From birth to six months of age, your baby is learning to move all the parts of his mouth through an ingenious system of reflexes. One of the first you will notice is the rooting reflex, where your baby turns his head toward any touch on his cheek. Mother Nature is helping your baby locate the breast for nursing, until he begins to associate the smell and feel of his mother's breast with food. As the reflex begins to fade, baby has enough experience to purposefully turn toward the breast when hungry, becoming quite the food-finding expert by three months of age.

How is it that babies know instinctively to suckle on the breast? It's a reflex activated when touch receptors on the back of the throat and on the lips detect something entering the mouth.[18] This is why lactation consultants will encourage moms to put as much breast in baby's mouth as possible, so that all the receptors receive the suckling signal and baby achieves and maintains a good latch. Suckling is the beginning stage of learning to suck and involves a forward-backward movement, like steady waves rolling onto a beach. (We'll discuss sucking in the next chapter.) Once your baby is actively engaged in suckling, you'll notice a rhythm to the way he suckles, swallows, and breathes. Swallowing is also reflexive and remains that way throughout life. Older toddlers can learn "how, what, and why" we swallow, but they never lose the ability to swallow reflexively. We even swallow while sleeping!

Coach Mel's Tip:
Tongue-ties and Upper Lip Ties

If your baby is having trouble latching or sucking, or having other feeding challenges, it may be because of an unde-tected tongue-tie (ankyloglossia) or upper lip tie (ULT). Tongue-ties are not always obvious and some require close examination by an experienced professional. Tongue-ties don't always look alike but are defined by the International Affiliation of Tongue-tie Profes-sionals as "an embryological remnant of tissue in the midline between the undersurface of the tongue and the floor of the mouth that restricts normal tongue movement. Tongue-tie can thereby adversely affect infant feeding, eating, chewing, speech, and even breathing if left untreated for too long."[18] Because there are so many variations or "looks" of a tongue-tie, we recommend consult-ing your pediatrician who can refer you for an assessment with the appro-priate professional. The ULT also restricts movement when the v-shaped tissue (the frenum) that attaches the upper lip to the upper gums inhibits upper lip movement. Babies need good mobility of the upper lip in order to latch and breast-feed, eat food off a spoon, and manipulate food for chewing and swallowing.

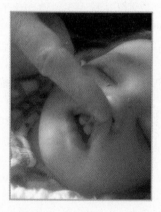

Another reflex that will one day help baby learn to eat is the bite reflex. When you put your finger on a newborn's gums, he'll gnaw on your finger. Baby is learning from that reflex for several months, as well as exercising muscles that he will one day use for talking and eating, until the reflex disappears by age one.[19] Put your finger in too far and baby will gag, which is a protective reflex that is stimulated when there is an unfamiliar or over-stimulating touch behind the broad tip of the baby's tongue.

All these reflexes are preparing your baby to explore purees and other solid foods, discussed in our next chapter.

Coach Mel's Tip:
Don't Feed Baby in the Car Seat

Try your best to avoid feeding your baby in a car seat or infant carrier. The shape of these seats puts baby's hips at an angle, where the pelvis is tilted back (like slumping in a chair), and will put pressure on the Lower Esophageal Sphincter (LES). Increased pressure means more frequent refluxing, even if the baby isn't spitting up. This "silent" reflux can cause damage over time as the stomach acid begins to irritate and inflame the esophagus. Holding baby for bottle-feeding is important for esophageal health and is vital for parent-child bonding.

Many babies often have gastroesophageal reflux (GER), meaning they frequently spit up. The opening from the esophagus to the stomach is known as the lower esophageal sphincter (LES), a tight band of muscle tissue that relaxes and constricts in order to hold the contents of the stomach (including stomach acid) until it empties into the intestines below. While many babies are occasional "happy spitters," some frequently experience GER when the sphincter opens too often. Causes include low muscle tone and an immature nervous system sending signals to the LES at inopportune times. These factors (and more) are frequently related to premature birth, although they can be found in full-term babies too. Signs that your baby is refluxing stomach acid to the point of discomfort include, but are not limited to: weight loss, arching during and after feedings, coughing, increased fussiness throughout the day, and needing small, frequent feedings day and night. Over time, babies who suffer from frequent discomfort may be diagnosed with gastroesophageal reflux disease (GERD), which may be managed with medications in addition to strategies related to positioning and frequency and volume of feeding. Mothers who are breast-feeding may need to follow a special diet free of suspected allergens if baby is spitting up frequently. Specialized formula that has proteins broken down to aid in digestion may also be an option to ensure that baby not only continues to grow and thrive, but also doesn't relate feeding to discomfort. We don't want babies to associate eating with pain.

How to Guide Your Child: Oral Motor Skills

Mother Nature has provided reflexes to introduce each lesson, but you are the true teacher as you guide your child through the steps to successful eating, even before introducing solid foods. As baby experiences oral reflexes in action, she'll learn to make the same movements intentionally. You can help her by doing the following:

1. Seek professional guidance. Don't hesitate to seek guidance from a lactation consultant, even if breast-feeding appears to be going well at first. They are experts in preventing issues from arising, which may later impact your baby's ability to gain weight and grow. Before an issue arises, connect with an expert to teach you tips for successful breast-feeding.

2. Introduce the bottle this way. For bottle-feeding, take advantage of baby's natural suckling reflex by gently yet firmly touching baby's lips with the bottle's nipple. Roll the nipple into baby's mouth and press the nipple on the central groove of the tongue (the line that divides the tongue into a left and right side). This gentle pressure will initiate the suckling reflex and baby will curl the sides of his tongue around the nipple.[20]

3. Offer gentle cheek support. Some babies benefit from gentle cheek support: using your thumb and index finger, as pictured here. This provides just enough stability for the jaw, lips, and tongue to operate effectively and decreases fatigue. For additional chin support, place your longest finger just under baby's chin bone. Your finger should still move up and down a bit as baby sucks and not restrict the movement. Be sure not to use too much pressure as this can change the force of the milk flow within the baby's mouth.

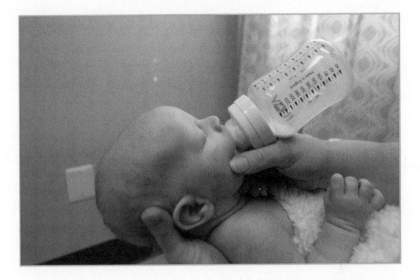

4. Consider the size of your baby's mouth. Use a nipple size and shape that fits your baby's mouth. Most feeding therapists prefer a rounded or cylindrical nipple because it encourages the tongue to curl up on the sides. However, there are exceptions to this rule. Begin with a rounded nipple and if your baby is having significant difficulty, ask your pediatrician to refer you to a feeding therapist.

5. Compare bottle nipples. If the milk flow is too slow, baby may fatigue more quickly (and take in fewer calories). If the milk flow is too fast and makes feeding too easy, baby may not exercise the muscles essential for eating solid foods and talking. Most importantly, if the flow is too fast, baby may lose coordination and cough, and/or lose control of liquid from the corners of his mouth, making feeding a very unpleasant experience. For some babies this increases their risk of aspiration (breathing in liquid).

The key is to watch for baby's signs of coordination, rhythm, and comfort. Most full-term infants and older babies can finish their bottles while maintaining a steady pace with occasional breaks for burping. Bottle nipples also break down with repeated washing and the flow will change over time. Don't wait for obvious signs of wear and tear. Replace bottle nipples every two months and consider advancing to the next stage as baby's skills improve.

6. Pick the perfect pacifier. The shape of baby's pacifier, should you decide to use one, is important and should mimic the bottle nipple if you're bottle-feeding. A popular pacifier used in many hospital nurseries is the Avent Soothie pacifier, which follows American Academy of Pediatrics (AAP) guidelines[21] and is constructed of a single piece, for safety. As baby grows, she made need a larger pacifier to ensure that she cannot place the entire thing in her mouth. Like bottle nipples, pacifiers need to be replaced frequently to ensure that no small pieces accidently break off. Don't worry, we'll help you wean baby off the pacifier by eighteen months (outlined in chapter 5), so if you choose to use one now to soothe your baby, it's OK! Pacifiers are especially helpful for calming babies who are sensitive to environmental stimuli. Plus, providing your baby with a pacifier while she is sleeping has been found to reduce the risk of SIDS and is recommended by the AAP.[22]

7. Limit dream feeding. While babies may fall asleep occasionally toward the end of breast- or bottle-feeding, it's important that they are awake for most of the feeding so that they can learn from the suckling reflex. Dream feeding, or feeding a baby while he is partially asleep, is possible because between birth and six months, the suckling reflex is automatic. But if baby is taking most of the feeding while even partially asleep, he has very limited opportunities to learn to suck on his own. It's not unusual for Coach Mel to be called into a home to help a seven-month-old baby who has "forgotten" how to suck, because he had been fed in his sleep for much of his young life. As the suckling reflex integrates and baby must now suck purposefully on his own, he has significant difficulty initiating and maintaining the rhythm and motor planning necessary for suck-swallow-breathe coordination. In simpler terms, they just can't figure it out because they were asleep during the learning process.

Dr. Yum's Tip: Look for Signs of Fullness

While babies are learning to regulate their intake, notice the cues that may indicate they are full. In the first few days, babies may take only one ounce or so at a time, but soon they will be able to handle more as they become more alert and their stomach capacity increases. A general rule to go by: Once they get into the swing of feeding, most full-term newborns feed "two to three ounces every two to three hours" (formula-fed babies may stretch this interval out to four hours). However, some babies may need more or less volume and a longer or shorter frequency depending on their size, their stomach capacity, whether they have a tendency to spit up, etc.

Watch for signs that your baby is full, like pulling away from the breast or bottle, turning his head, or becoming distracted. Signs your baby may need more food are crying or smacking his lips at end of the feed. Keep in mind that the day baby is born, his stomach capacity is equivalent to a marble (5–7 ml) and that by day three it has grown to the size of a ping-pong ball (22–27 ml). It slowly begins to stretch over time, and when baby is ten days old, his stomach capacity is similar to an extra-large egg (60–81 ml).[23]

8. Listen to baby. Although it's helpful to have guidelines on how much to feed your baby, feeding is truly a dance between parent and child. Over the first few months, you'll begin to distinguish between baby's various cries: "I'm hungry," "I'm tired," or "I need to be held." In addition to cries, try to observe and identify baby's preliminary cues that she is hungry, which may include rooting, bringing hands to mouth and sucking, and/or having an anticipatory, alert facial expression. Cues that baby is full or needs a break in feeding include baby pausing during feeding, turning away from the nipple, slowing down her pace, and/or squirming.

For more tips on cue-based feeding, even if your child was

born full-term, take a minute to read "A Closer Look: The Premature Baby," on page 43.

9. Understand that sucking has many purposes. These include nutrition, calming (non-nutritive sucking), and organization of the sensory system. Plus, sucking encourages proper palate formation in breast-fed babies. Learning to suckle begins in the womb, and it's not unusual to see baby sucking on his thumb during an ultrasound as early as twenty-one weeks of gestation! Babies who learn to suck their thumbs in the womb are in a natural flexed position where the spine is slightly curved and the hands are at midline, close to the mouth. As baby grows in the cramped quarters of the uterus, the thumb is near the mouth most of the time, and baby can't help but get lots of practice before entering the world!

10. Sucking for comfort. Over the next six months, frequency of feeds may decrease while their volume increases. It's easy to misinterpret a baby's reflexes as a cue to eat. When you feel like your baby is full but still wants to suck, try offering comfort (perhaps with a pacifier or your finger) instead of more milk. A typical six-month-old may take six to eight ounces of milk every five to six hours, with longer stretches of sleep at night. Establishing these longer stretches at night is important to protect baby's newly emerging teeth from decay, or "milk bottle caries," which can occur from frequent night feedings (nursing or bottle-feeding).

 Visualizing the capacity of your baby's stomach using the "belly balls" model noted above is helpful, but being sensitive to your child's fullness cues is also an important parenting habit to establish early in life. Maintaining this sensitivity is one of the key parenting strategies for teaching your children lifelong healthy eating habits.

Thumb, Pacifier, or Neither?

When considering "thumb, paci, or neither" for your infant, there are always pros and cons. It's easy for an unborn baby in the tight space of the uterus to reach her thumb, but during the first month of life the newborn will need to be swaddled in order to keep her thumb near her mouth. A pacifier is sometimes more readily available, if it doesn't fall out. As baby grows and it's time to wean from sucking on a thumb or paci, it's much easier to throw out a pacifier than a thumb.

When it comes to feeding, the most common concern is how sucking will impact a child's oral motor skills and interest in food. The solution is to limit pacifier and thumb sucking to bedtime by age nine months. By eighteen months, we recommend weaning baby completely from the pacifier and/or thumb so that it doesn't affect palate formation and dentition,[24] which will have a direct impact on feeding skills.

Coach Mel's Tip:
Parenting Proactively with Tube Feedings

Many parents encounter an unexpected feeding detour with their infants, who, for a variety of medical reasons, may not be able to breast- or bottle-feed. A nasogastric (NG) tube, which is a narrow, flexible tube inserted through the nose (or sometimes the mouth), may be necessary for liquid nutrition. Some babies may require a feeding tube surgically inserted through the abdominal wall (one common type is known as a gastrostomy tube, or g-tube) until they can learn to eat orally. Although it may take some time to learn to eat by mouth, it's important for parents to support their child's learning via the reflexes. With the guidance of a feeding therapist, take advantage of baby's reflexes, which provide repetitive practice for her. A feeding therapist can assist parents in preparing the baby for food experiences by practicing with non-food items before the reflexes disappear.

Although it's heartbreaking for parents when their child experiences feeding challenges, it's comforting to know that there is a lot parents can do to help their baby learn from the oral reflexes. Even when using a feeding tube, these first six months are vital opportunities for successful oral motor development through proactive parenting.

Cognitive Skills Related to Feeding

By three months of age, baby is following objects with his eyes with ease and anticipating food when he sees the breast or bottle. By six months of age, he understands that if he drops a toy, it will fall. He intentionally activates basic cause-and-effect toys (for example, pushing a button to hear a sound) because he's learned that if he does one action, a specific reaction will occur.

These cognitive milestones prepare baby for future feeding skills, such as anticipating the food on a spoon or the taste of the squished avocado that he holds in his tiny fist. These early experiences lead to later events like dropping his cracker over the edge of the high chair tray, just so he can feed the dog. It's all part of the developmental process of learning to eat!

THE PREMATURE INFANT'S MOTOR SKILLS

- Parenting with Patience: Why the early-term or premature babies need extra time for feeding skills
- Gross and fine motor development on its own special timeline

We have a special place in our hearts for premature babies, who often need more specific attention in the first two years of life. They come into the world small and fragile, but so many of them grow and thrive to the point that no one could imagine how tiny they once were. Parenting with patience is essential to help these little babies reach their potential.

A CLOSER LOOK
The Premature Baby

The American Academy of Obstetrics and Gynecology has recognized that the "previously-used classification of 'term gestation' of 37–42 weeks" did not reflect the varying outcomes and maturity of this wide group. They recently redefined preterm and term gestations in the following way:

Early-term: 37 0/7 through 38 6/7 weeks of gestation
Full-term: 39 0/7 through 40 6/7 weeks of gestation
Late-term: 41 0/7 through 41 6/7 weeks of gestation
Post-term: 42 0/7 weeks of gestation and beyond[25]

How does this new terminology relate to the way that babies feed? "Early-term" reminds us that we need to be patient while we wait for babies to establish full-term feeding skills. A full-term baby may have an easier time learning to latch and breast-feed effectively, while the early-term baby might take a bit more time to establish a nursing pattern.

Preemie Gross Motor Skills

Infants who are born before thirty-seven weeks of gestation often have unique gross motor development challenges. Their primary focus is on breathing and growing. Preemies spend much of the day sleeping, but as they mature, they have periods of alertness where they can begin to practice gross motor control. Yet, even a baby born at thirty-six weeks of gestation does not have the same muscle tone or hold his body in the same position as a baby born at forty weeks.

Each week, new progress is made and every preemie is evaluated by considering his developmental age, not his gestational age. In fact, preemies are given a full two years before they are expected to meet the same developmental milestones as babies born full-term. Thus, a baby born four weeks early is not expected to sit up on his own at six months, but is given an extra four weeks to achieve that goal. Consequently, because all feeding skills are a developmental process, your baby may be ready for solid foods four weeks later than you might expect. No matter what his age, every baby is unique, and your pediatrician will be keeping close tabs on your preemie to ensure that he continues to grow, thrive, and move to the next steps when he is ready, regardless of the calendar.

 Dr. Yum's Tip: Your Preemie's Adjusted Age
When a baby is born prematurely, development and growth may not follow those of other babies that are born at term around the same birthday. To correct for that difference, pediatricians use a corrected or adjusted age, which is the infant's actual age minus the number of weeks or months of prematurity. For example, a ten-month-old baby who was born two months early may have the growth and development of an eight-month-old, which would be considered their adjusted age. Many pediatricians will continue to correct a child's age when assessing growth and development until about age two. So, a six-month-old preemie may not be expected to sit up on his own until he is in the world for eight months, to allow some "catch-up" time. Some premature babies may take a longer or shorter period of time to adjust to their chronological age.

Preemie Fine Motor Skills and Oral Motor Skills

Learning to coordinate the mouth for future feedings is an early fine motor skill—and oral motor skill. As with many skills, premature babies may take additional time to feed well. In the case of the extremely premature baby, she may receive nutrition by intravenous (IV) feeding or a nutrition tube. It's typically inserted into a larger vein, bypassing the baby's immature stomach until it's ready to receive feedings. Once a baby can receive feedings by mouth, suckle and swallow reflexes still may not be mature enough to manage oral feedings. A tiny feeding tube may be inserted into the stomach through the nose or mouth to provide calories, as noted in Coach Mel's tip on page 41. Eventually, as the baby becomes stronger and bigger, feedings by mouth may be gradually introduced.

Preemies will not have the same oral motor skills as a full-term baby. Their reflexes and motor control are still developing, and now, the sensory system is being exposed to a very different world than the dark, warm comfort of the womb. The staff of the neonatal intensive care unit (NICU) will teach parents strategies that support baby's development and respect the preemie's immature and delicate sensory system. And the most important thing to remember is that growing takes time and that each baby grows at his own pace. Thus, preemies may begin their feeding journey with gavage (tube) feedings rather than oral feeds, because they aren't capable of breast- or bottle-feedings yet . . . but they will be soon! Each baby sets her own pace while parents and NICU staff gently guide her on the path to breast- and/or bottle-feeding.

As with babies of any age, by parenting mindfully, you can learn to read your baby's cues. Consider all behaviors meaningful, even baby's level of alertness. This is especially important for the premature infant, who is still learning to regulate various stages of alertness that are much easier to control after forty weeks of gestation. Behavioral states may range from *deep sleep* to *crying*, both easy to detect. But the states that lie in the middle of the spectrum take a bit of practice to interpret. *Light sleep* or *rapid eye movement (REM) sleep* may appear to be a time to rouse your baby if you need to feed him in order to maintain a feeding schedule for growth. But otherwise, allow him to rest during periods of light sleep. You'll find most preterm infants are in light sleep throughout their day. Resting can include "kangaroo care," where baby is placed on your or your partner's chest and covered with a blanket for added warmth. Hospital staff will assist you with your first kangaroo care experience, typically in an oversized, reclining chair in the nursery. Research shows that

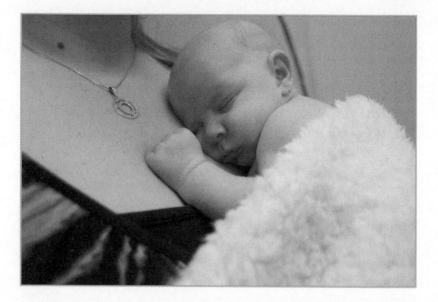

the warmth of your body heat, the sound of your heartbeat, and your love will help baby grow, even while the two of you doze together.[26]

Other states of arousal that you will observe include *drowsy, quiet alert,* and *active alert.* Quiet alert differs from active alert and is the perfect time to interact more socially with your baby. For preemies or babies sensitive to various stimuli, including movement, this is a time to keep your interactions soft with slow and steady movements. Even baby's vestibular system is attempting to take in new information and react appropriately, so quiet movements through space are important. If baby becomes over-stimulated, you'll lose the quiet alert state and baby may shift to a more protective state such as light sleep. Active alert can also signal a baby that is overstimulated, and you'll notice breathing becoming irregular, a loss in focus, and overreaction to your attempts to connect with him.

Ask staff in the NICU to help you observe and respond appropriately to these six behavioral states, because your baby will continue to exhibit these at home for many months to come.

PAYTON'S STORY:
Getting Back on Track

It's not uncommon for babies to have feeding challenges, especially if born early and/or with medical issues. Those babies need to focus on one thing: breathing. Feeding is secondary, at best. Learning to coordinate sucking, swallowing, and breathing is an advanced skill that even some full-term babies have trouble with at first. Although Coach Mel's role is to help boost those skills over time, babies set their own pace. It's a lesson that so many kids have taught Coach Mel along the way.

One memorable little teacher was baby Payton, born early-term. One month later, Payton had extensive abdominal surgery on her stomach and intestines, her appendix removed, a hernia repaired, and a g-tube placed in her abdomen. Payton needed to recover from major surgery and learn to drink from a bottle again.

It was an unexpected detour for her mom and dad, who were already parenting an eager eater, Payton's big sister, now three. The road ahead seemed very, very long. Her mother expressed her feelings of urgency: "In the back of my mind, I knew that this would be a long journey, but I didn't exactly know how long or what it would entail and I wanted to know *now*! Everyone in the hospital kept telling me that Payton would do this at her own pace ('Payton's Pace') but I didn't want to wait." Parenting patiently is the hardest when life throws you a curveball. You just want to get to your intended destination . . . immediately.

Payton's mother, father, and Coach Mel worked as a team to coax Payton back to bottle-feeding, then learning to eat solids, and finally, to removing the g-tube. Coach Mel tries to help parents understand the difference between setting goals and setting expectations. Therapeutic goals are clear targets or objectives. Expectations feel more passionate and are based on hope, anticipation, and beliefs.

As Payton's mom put it, "As a parent, when you have a child with any challenge, you have expectations for them that are based on your emotions, including sadness, anger, denial, and/ or hope." During their first feeding session together, Coach Mel asked her what she asks every parent just starting out in this process: "Tell me what you want for your child." Peyton's mom answered, "I want her to eat birthday cake on her first birthday," and then she stated it clearly once again, with tears in her eyes, just to ensure that Coach Mel understood. "She's *going* to eat birthday cake on her first birthday!"

Expectations are very emotional. As time went on, Payton taught all of us to respect her own pace of development. She did indeed have birthday cake on her first birthday, and a month or so later, the g-tube was removed. But she continued with feeding therapy for a few more months to polish those gross and fine motor skills that are so necessary to eat a variety of foods. She would do it at Payton's pace and we were just along for the ride.[27]

4

FIRST STEPS
Six to Eight Months
and on "Solid" Ground

Hooray! Your baby is ready for the adventure of solid foods. From six to nine months there is a period of rapid and exciting food exploration. Even though your new little eater has been feeding since birth, the transition to solid foods opens up a whole new world of tastes and textures. For weeks, you may have noticed your baby interested in what you're eating. Now he gets to try some of those foods for himself! Just like breast- or bottle-feeding, learning to eat solids starts with understanding basic child development in babies this age, beginning with gross motor development. This advancement in gross motor skills also coincides with fine motor and oral motor skills progress—it's all connected! Plus, baby's brain is taking in information, cataloging it, and creating memories related to food experiences. We are stepping onto "solid" ground—in more ways than one!

GROSS MOTOR SKILL DEVELOPMENT

- Why proper positioning in the high chair can make all the difference!
- Parent Bravely: A few bumps are part of the journey
- Parent Proactively: Set your child up for success

From six to eight months, there are so many marvelous gross motor advances. By six months, you may notice your baby has more truncal support and head control. His head was once wobbly and needed your support, but now it's steadier when he is in a seated position. When you help lift your baby from lying to sitting using his arms, he is now likely to have enough strength for his head to lead the rest of his body instead of lagging behind, like when he was a newborn.

By six months of age, most babies are ready to begin sitting up on their own. They may transfer objects from hand to hand and have a purposeful grasp. By seven months, a baby may lift his head and torso off the ground when he is on his tummy, in preparation for crawling. He may begin to stand holding on to a support. By the end of the eighth month, most babies can get themselves to a seated position and can pull themselves up to stand. They start to find unique and interesting ways to navigate around a room, so get those baby gates up! All the strength they are developing will make it possible for them to sit in a stable position and begin accepting solid foods safely.

How to Guide Your Child: Gross Motor Skills

To help your baby start sitting on her own, place her in a seated position with her legs widely spaced apart. Bring both her arms in front of her and plant them firmly between her legs, like a tripod. The support of her arms will ground her as she gets used to this position.

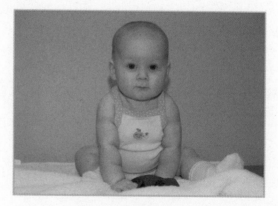

Spend time on the ground with your baby, letting her try this position. Gradually test her core strength by handing her an object and letting her balance with one hand as a tripod, and then eventually with no hands. Be sure to alternate placing the toy at midline (in line with baby's nose) and on either side of midline. This way, babies don't learn to favor one hand (Remember, we don't expect hand dominance until after age three) and they also learn to cross over midline with the opposite hand. It's important that babies develop both sides of their brain.

As your baby gains strength, stability, and coordination, you'll begin to see her reaching across midline with her right hand to find a toy (or eventually, some yummy steamed broccoli!) on the left side of her high chair tray.

PARENT BRAVELY Letting your baby gain independence can sometimes mean letting go of fear. When allowing babies to explore a space, always supervise. Try to remove any objects that could pose a danger, but know that you can't anticipate everything. Getting an occasional bump on the head from a soft surface when trying to stand is part of the process of learning to walk and will be the first of many bumps and bruises he will have as he gains more independence.

The first step to learning to eat solids, even purees, is being correctly positioned in the feeding chair. The ideal position is to have baby sit upright, with some added support around her, in a chair that has a back—not a cube-shaped "booster seat." If your baby can't quite sit up on her own, you can let her lean back slightly in a feeding chair that is intended to recline. Be sure that your baby is supported at the hips so that she doesn't slide forward and slump. Try sitting back in a chair and slumping your posture: It's not easy to chew and swallow in that position.

Here's how to position your baby:

1. Begin at her hips. There is an old saying among feeding therapists, "What happens at the hips, you see on the lips." In essence, it means that fine motor skills are always dependent on gross motor stability, and your baby's fulcrum is her hips. The *angle* of the hips is important. Make sure your baby's pelvis is tilted slightly forward to provide a base for her trunk. When the pelvis is tilted backward, it leads to that undesirable slumped posture described earlier, throwing off the entire alignment of the trunk, neck, and head.

2. Add bolsters. To ensure that all of baby's body parts align above the hips, roll up some hand towels into tube-shaped bolsters and place them to the left and right of baby's ribcage. You may want to place a narrow bolster under baby's knees for added stability and to help keep his back against the high chair. Be sure that any extra supports don't interfere with buckling the high chair's safety straps. Always use those to secure your child.

3. Place baby's feet on a footrest. Next, consider what's happening below the hips. Once baby has grown to the point where his knees can bend over the edge of the seat, it is vital that his little feet are on a footrest. While most high chairs come with a footrest, it takes many months before baby's toes can reach it. Feel free to grab a cracker box and duct tape it to the footrest in order to raise it up to meet your baby's shoes. If you've ever had to sit on a bar stool with your feet dangling, you can relate to how tiring it can be! We all need something under our feet for stability, and babies need it even more because they're still developing the trunk muscles that keep an adult upright on that bar stool.

 Most parents are surprised to learn that something as simple as positioning a child a specific way in the feeding chair can make a world of difference. Parenting proactively means setting your child up for success by anticipating and preparing for the next developmental milestone.

4. Check the tray. With baby sitting upright, check to make sure the high chair tray (or tabletop if the chair is pushed up to your family table) is at the bottom of baby's breastbone. You may need to add a folded towel under the high chair cover to boost baby just a bit. Her elbows should fit comfortably on the tray without her having to hunch her shoulders. This position provides extra stability for learning to rake up or hold first finger foods. Baby may also grab the spoon as you feed her softer foods, and that's terrific! We'll cover more about self-spoon-feeding in the next chapter, but for now, baby will enjoy holding the spoon and use it mostly for dipping, mouthing, swatting, and banging.

 Coach Mel's Tip:
Cushion Your Baby with Shelf Liner!
Buy several rolls of spongy, waffle-weave shelf liner at the dollar store. Not only can it be rolled up to serve as bolsters, but also it provides just the right amount of traction for little bottoms to sit on. By adding a small square of shelf liner to the seat of the high chair cushion, your baby will stick in one spot, keeping the pelvis at just the right tilt and preventing the hips from sliding forward. Wrap a little extra piece around the footrest so tiny feet stick, too.

FINE MOTOR SKILL DEVELOPMENT

- Whether purees or solids, little hands need to get messy
- How babies develop the pincer grasp
- Parenting with Patience: The importance of waiting
- Baby-led weaning: Making the best choice for you and your child
- Parenting Bravely: Gagging vs. choking

By six months, babies are reaching and grabbing objects and may even pass them back to you. They may be able to "rake" objects toward themselves with their hands. By seven to eight months, a thumb-finger grasp may be forming, although not as delicate as the pincer grasp you will see at twelve months, which uses the very tips of the fingers. Instead, your baby may grab things with the thumb and side of the fingers. Still, these skills are enough to allow babies to pick up food and feed themselves, one of the concepts of baby-led weaning, a feeding trend covered later in this chapter.

 The feeling of compassion, in essence, is truly about reciprocity. Putting yourself in your child's shoes allows you to parent both respectfully *and* effectively. For many parenting challenges, a respectful and caring approach can help guide the child while supporting her unique spirit.

How to Guide Your Child: Fine Motor Skills

Once your child is sitting on her own or with a bit of support and you have her properly positioned in her high chair, she is ready to begin more independent feeding. This stage of the game is all about providing a variety of safe foods for her to try, engaging with her as she eats, and letting her get messy as she explores new foods.

Babies can begin the process of both spoon- and finger-feeding between the ages of five and six months, using both purees and soft, safe foods. Why? Because this is when babies acquire better lip control and movement as they suck the puree off a parent's finger, their own hands, or a spoon. When babies bite soft pieces of safe foods, they are learning via their rhythmic bite reflex. If the food is placed on the gums where we will one day see molars, a rotary chew pattern will begin to emerge over time, thanks to reflexive patterns that soon become purposeful movements.[28] Remember, feeding is a developmental process and *both* purees and finger-feeding facilitate the progression of skills.

Finger-feeding is the perfect opportunity for your little foodie to practice his pincer grasp, where he engages the tip of his thumb and forefinger to pick up pea-sized foods, such as halved blueberries and cereal. (A washable mat under the high chair tray is a must!)

At about six months, your child will begin to rake up objects by using his whole hand and curling all four fingers around the desired item. Letting go of the food can be tricky. You may see your child use his mouth to grab the food from his fists. Slowly, over the next two months, the pincer grasp will begin to emerge. This is also the time that children have enough trunk stability to sit in a high chair and focus on this new skill. Typically, by the end of baby's first year, she has perfected the pincer grasp! At that time, you will see your child begin to pick up small pieces of food and place them in her mouth with more precision and, thankfully, less mess. (See chapter 5 for parenting strategies on mastering the pincer grasp.)

You can support the natural progression of finger-feeding by offering soft foods or foods that melt in the mouth, such as a buttery cracker. It's relatively easy to grasp and mouth until a soft, mushy piece falls into his mouth. Over time, a baby will develop his ability to grade his jaw movement and truly bite into the cracker in a controlled, even manner. As his skills improve, offer pea-sized pieces of soft foods that expose your child to a variety of tastes, safe temperatures, and textures. Small, cold blueberries cut in half, warm, buttery pieces of pasta or tofu, or cereal spritzed with apple juice are all good starter foods.

 Allow children to find their way on their own. When you observe your child struggling at first to pick up a small piece of cereal, resist the urge to pick it up for him. This practice is important for him to perfect his skills. Of course, if a real sense of frustration is developing, offer him some gentle help: placing the cereal on a less slippery surface like your hand, or guiding the cereal closer to his fingers. The next time, he may be able to do it himself and will delight in his accomplishment as he puts the cereal in his mouth. This principle of patience is the same one that you will use down the road when you wait for him to tie his shoes or snap a button. You may be tempted to jump in and help, and it may take a few moments of waiting, but the self-reliance he learns is worth the price!

CLOSER LOOK:
Baby-Led Weaning from a Developmental Perspective

Baby-led weaning (BLW) is a term coined by Gill Rapley and Tracey Murkett, coauthors of *Baby-Led Weaning: The Essential Guide to Introducing Solid Foods.* In a nutshell, BLW centers on the philosophy that babies are capable of reaching for food and putting it in their mouths at about six months of age. (Please note that "wean" is not referring to weaning from breast or bottle, but instead is a term commonly used in the United Kingdom for adding complementary foods to the baby's current diet of breast milk or formula.) The BLW model offers many advantages:

- BLW encourages parents to eat with their children, since everyone is eating the same food. In today's busy culture, it feels easier to many parents to feed the baby prior to the adult or family meal, and in BLW the thought is that jarred purees contribute to this habit. Please note that we think purees are important to the developmental process of feeding, but agree it's important to include baby at the table at an early age.

- BLW emphasizes that babies must be the ones to put the food in their mouths (we emphasize that feeding is a reciprocal and interactive activity). It's essential to encourage self-feeding because it allows kids to get messy. Babies are programmed to explore the world with all their senses, especially their hands and mouths, and often the two together! BLW notes that the time to begin self-feeding is at six months when baby can sit upright on her own. Of course, *every* child must have the gross motor stability to support fine motor skills, including reaching and raking for food and controlling their grasp to bring the food to the mouth. For children who have this capability, we feel comfortable with letting them mouth large pieces of food that will not snap off (or allow a solid chunk to fall into the mouth), in addition to short spoons and chewable toys for practicing the skills that will eventually lead to self-feeding.

- BLW follows the baby's cues, rather than the parent controlling the feeding via the spoon. Whether presenting food to your child by placing it on the high chair tray in front of them, directly on a spoon, or even mouth to mouth as done in some cultures, reading baby's cues for readiness is crucial. Like a beautiful, flowing conversation, feeding children is a reciprocal experience.[29]

- BLW encourages parents to become comfortable with gagging episodes and understand the difference between gagging and choking. Gagging and choking are two different experiences. Typically, an infant's gag reflex is triggered when the back three-quarters of the tongue is stimulated, but by the time a child reaches nine months of age, the reflex covers less area: the back third of the tongue. Eventually, the gag reflex shifts farther back, even more so as the child learns to tolerate the stimulation. Gagging is nature's way of protecting the airway, where true choking occurs.

- Choking happens when a food (or other substance) obstructs the airway and thus often has no sound or intermittent, odd sounds. Other signs of choking include gasping for breath, turning blue around the lips and beneath the eyes, and/or staring with an open mouth while drooling.

- Gagging is an uncomfortable sensation where the soft palate suddenly elevates, the jaw thrusts forward and down, and the back of the tongue lifts up and forward. It is not unusual for a child to vomit after gagging. In between the gags, the child is still able to breathe, cry, and make vocal noises. Gagging is an important built-in safety mechanism, but frequent gags and/or vomiting can lead to an aversion to food.[30]

If you would like to follow baby-led weaning principles, we stress the importance of reading baby's cues and monitoring her closely for safe feeding while supporting her through the developmental process of learning to eat, no matter what age. This includes proper positioning in the feeding chair for optimal stability and presenting only manageable pieces of solid foods, along with purees, that do not pose a choking hazard. And for children in feeding therapy, incorporating some aspects of BLW is dependent on that child's individual delays or challenges and where they are in the developmental process, regardless of chronological age.

 So many parents we encounter express that the fear of choking and gagging keeps them from letting their baby advance beyond smooth purees. Now that you know the difference, you can bravely navigate the introduction of solid foods with confidence.

ORAL MOTOR SKILL DEVELOPMENT

- How to use a baby spoon correctly
- No two spoons are alike—which to choose?
- Parenting Mindfully: That beautiful face!

Over the past six months, your baby has learned from her suckling reflex *how* to suck independently. She can initiate sucking at the breast or bottle on her own and maintain the pattern with ease. Today, that suckling reflex is beginning to fade, which is ideal timing for new skills like biting and chewing to be discovered! The tongue's tendency to move in a forward-backward pattern is a familiar movement for baby, and her first attempts at eating purees or squishy, soft foods may result in food spilling out over her lips. As she matures, the forward-back motion will disappear and baby will develop a "mature swallow pattern," which allows the food to stay inside the mouth and prevents spillage. Plus, with time, baby will learn how to propel the food backwards to be swallowed. That's why purees are often the first foods to be offered to baby: They are the easiest foods to suck off fingers or a spoon and then swallow. Purees are the bridge to learning to self-feed.

As baby becomes comfortable with soft foods, you'll notice that she'll begin to practice biting and "chewing" even though there are no teeth yet. Sometimes, the food appears to get spit out, but it's more likely that she is learning to control the new sensations and the food itself inside her mouth. Keep offering the food, gently and positively. It takes time for all of us to adjust to new foods and when it's your very first time, it takes many attempts to master it!

How to Guide Your Child: Oral Motor Skills

Where to start? Perhaps you've decided to start with purees, presented on a spoon. If you've visited your local baby goods aisle, the array of different feeding spoons can be overwhelming. Some spoons come with holes to allow liquid to drain and solids to stick. Other spoons are textured for those children who need more tactile input in their mouths in order to tell where the spoon is about to dump the food. Some spoons come with bendable "necks," so that parents can adjust the angle to facilitate better hand-to-mouth coordination.

Here's all you need to know to feed your six-month-old:

1. Choose a spoon that has a small, flat "bowl" to fit your baby's tiny mouth. The flatter surface ensures that you won't scoop up too much food, making it easier to swallow all at once, and it encourages your baby to close his lips on the spoon and suck off the puree.

2. Never scrape the top of the spoon on baby's upper gum line or the roof of his mouth. That will encourage him to push his tongue up onto the puree, and thrust forward in order to push (rather than suck) the food onto the back of his tongue. That tongue protusion needs to fade in order for baby to move on to more advanced textures.

3. You can also hand baby squishy foods, such as slices of avocado or soft baked apple with the skin removed. Handling the wet texture tells the brain what it might feel like in her mouth. Baby's fine motor skills are focusing on raking and squeezing, so plenty of soft sweet potato or creamy risotto on the high chair tray provides the perfect opportunity for lots of tactile input for wet, sticky foods that cling to fingers. Mouthing, biting, sucking on fingers, or sucking on spoons—these are all part of the process of learning to manage and enjoy solid foods.

 Be sure that you're facing your baby and gazing eye-to-eye while enjoying feeding time together. If you're tall, you may need to sit in a shorter chair when feeding baby. Just like breast- and bottle-feeding is a time for bonding, family mealtimes are, too! It starts here—face-to-face, eye-to-eye. Besides, who could resist that beautiful baby face? Baby can't resist yours either!

Cognitive Skills Related to Feeding

By six months of age, baby has developed a strong sense of object permanence, or the understanding that objects, animals, and humans still exist even though they may not be seen. Or they may be sensed in another way, such as hearing the cat meow. Peekaboo is now a favorite, predictable game, and anticipating the "Boo!" when you uncover your face is where baby finds the most delight. That's why you may hear baby giggle just before you make the big reveal.

Although he enjoyed peekaboo while learning how to play the game at age four to five months (he's so much more grown up now!) the cognitive shift at this age focuses on the consistency of the game itself. What you may not realize is that over time, you've been nurturing your child's social turn-taking or "reciprocity." That reciprocity is essential to future social interactions, including the social skills integral to family mealtimes.[31]

You're creating memories with your child. Baby is taking in information, comparing it to prior information, and then cataloging it in his brain. These first experiences with solid foods are the foundation for future acceptances of various tastes, textures, and even temperatures. Your social interactions during mealtimes contribute to those memories—so parent mindfully and joyfully! Every smile, every giggle, and every moment counts.

FOODS FOR YOUR GROWING BABY

- One meal for one family: Making baby food is easy!
- Methods for preparing baby food
- Which foods are best? How much? How often?

The Argument for Homemade Baby Food

One of the ways that you can prioritize healthy food is to make your own baby food. Making baby food is not hard, but it teaches us to slow down as parents and take time to make sure that our child is eating wholesome, lovingly prepared food. It also instantly brings your child into the rest of the family's eating experience. While you're eating baked sweet potatoes, your baby can eat a version of the same. There is no reason your baby can't enjoy the hearty stew that you have prepared. Your own table food with a few small adjustments can be made easily into baby food.

These concepts train parents that there is no "special" meal for kids, and trains children that they eat the same food as their parents. A family meal is shared by *everyone* in the family, including the newest eater. Since you and your baby will be eating much of the same food, the kitchen tools you need will be pretty much the same. Resist the urge to spend money on fancy baby food systems. Your baby will be past the stage of pureed food before you know it!

One of the other great perks about homemade baby food is how easily you can customize recipes. For instance, babies have an innate preference for sweeter foods and a distaste for overly bitter foods until they are exposed to them repeatedly. To get a baby used to a bitter food, you may combine it with something sweeter. There are no rules here! Combine butternut squash with Brussels sprouts or asparagus with applesauce. Your baby does not know what the conventional combinations are, so try interesting flavors together and see how she likes it. Have fun trying these combinations yourself, too!

When you make our own baby food you can also adjust the texture to your baby's needs. Leave a bit more texture in one day and see how she responds. Too lumpy? Give it a few more whirls in the blender and try more texture when she seems ready.

Baby food made at home is also considerably less expensive than buying jars of baby food, and because it's less watered down, it is more flavorful. Remember, after six months of waiting to start solids, your baby is ready for even more flavor! Also, making your own food gives you the option of buying local, seasonal and/or organic ingredients that might be in line with how the rest of your family eats. There is nothing wrong with store-bought baby food. It can serve as an option for on-the-go feeding and when time is scarce. But the flavors and experience of making baby food cannot be matched by the store-bought versions.

When Dr. Yum taught her first baby food class in the kitchen at her practice, she set out to show parents how easy making baby food can be. Little did she realize the ripple effect that cooking for a baby can have in a family. A mom and dad from her practice came to the class with their six-month-old baby and learned some techniques for feeding solids to babies. At their next checkup, Dr. Yum was eager to hear how this baby was doing with his eating habits and what foods he was enjoying. Mom reported that her son was eagerly eating many new fruits and vegetables, and then added, "Guess who else is discovering how good vegetables are?" She pointed to her husband.

He blushed and said, "Yeah, I never really liked veggies, but now that we are making all this food for the baby I'm trying some of these foods and realizing I really like squash and sweet potatoes. Who knew?" The beautiful thing about learning to parent in the kitchen is that while we teach our kids great eating habits, there can be so many opportunities to better ourselves. Starting solid foods is that first time you are *preparing* food for your baby and sharing food with him. This is the foundation for the family culture of wellness you're building and one of the first big steps toward adventurous eating.

Starter Foods and Methods of Preparing Baby Food

The first thing parents ask when starting solid foods is, "What is the best first food to start with?" The pendulum swings back and forth on this topic, and it seems that whether you offer meats, veggies, or cereal first, most babies seem to experience first foods easily. When thinking about raising an adventurous eater, consider introducing complex tastes from the beginning. Rice cereal used to be the go-to first food, but in fact, that is probably one of the blandest foods around (see more about rice cereal in box below). However, what is nice about cereals (preferably whole grain) is they can be made to a very thin consistency with breast milk, formula, or water for the very first feedings. As you prepare other foods like fruits and vegetables, use formula, breast milk, or water to achieve the consistency you want when mashing or blending. If you're steaming, reserve the water in the pot to thin foods, too.

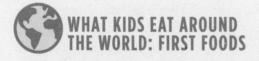

WHAT KIDS EAT AROUND THE WORLD: FIRST FOODS

It's clear that the traditional American first food of white rice cereal is a flavorless and uninspired choice compared to the variety of first foods seen in other cultures. Dr. Alan Greene, a well-known pediatrician and author, started a "White Out" campaign to educate families on giving babies alternatives to white cereal. On his website, drgreene.com, he says, "For the past fifty years the majority of babies in the United States have been given white rice cereal for their very first bite of baby food. It's a refined carb that babies don't need. White rice cereal is the number one food source of calories until about eleven months old. Let's reverse a half century of habit."[33] We agree that a better choice for first foods can be real whole foods prepared at home.

Here is a sampling of first foods that are offered across the globe. Seeing how different these traditions are, we can understand that there are so many ways to transition babies to solid foods.

JAMAICA: Pureed tropical fruits like banana, mango, custard apple (a native Jamaican fruit), and papaya are often the first fruits for Jamaican babies.

NIGERIA: Babies in Nigeria are often fed "gari," a soft flour made of fermented cassava root. The flour is then made into a dough or porridge. Babies are also fed yams and okra, as well as tripe for protein.

CHINA: "Congee," or rice porridge, is one of the first foods that Chinese babies may eat around four to six months. Rice is cooked with a lot of water or stock for a long period of time until the grains break down and soften. They may add vegetables or fish for extra flavoring and nutrients.

UNITED STATES: Some first foods for Inuit babies in Alaska are seaweed and muktuk (seal blubber). By nine months of age, berries, herbs, and meats like caribou are introduced.

Steaming and poaching are great cooking methods. To steam, use a small amount of water in a pot and use a steamer basket to hold the food inside it. Cover the pot and steam until tender. Poaching is another method of cooking in a small amount of water. This is a great way to cook chicken, which can then be pureed with soft foods. To poach a chicken breast, place it in the bottom of a pan and cover it with water. Bring to a boil and then simmer for at least eight minutes. Check it every few minutes until done. If you're unsure, insert a thermometer into the thickest part and cook until it reads 165°F. For both poaching and steaming, reserve the leftover water to thin foods to a desired consistency.

Roasting foods can be a nice way to soften them and bring out their natural sweetness. Most foods can be roasted at 350 to 400°F, but watch them and use a fork to test if the food is soft enough to smash or puree. A favorite baby recipe among our patients has been roasted bananas and sweet potatoes. Use water, breast milk, formula, or other soft foods to thin to the desired consistency. Some foods, like berries, may be best introduced by gently cooking or roasting them, and after many exposures can be diced raw. Once foods are prepared, blend them using a mini food processor or blender to get them smooth and soft, and add liquid to achieve the right consistency.

If you find yourself with leftovers, you can freeze these in a covered ice cube tray. Once frozen, keep them in a freezer-safe bag for three to six months. Reheat gently for homemade baby food on busy nights when there is no time to cook.

WHAT YOU WILL NEED TO START MAKING BABY FOOD

Baking sheet for roasting

Blender or mini food processor

Pot with steamer basket

Covered ice cube tray (optional)

FOODS YOU CAN STEAM OR POACH

Apples

Carrots

Cauliflower

Chicken

Pears

Peaches

Plums

Summer squash

Sweet peas

Zucchini

FOODS YOU CAN ROAST:

Apples

Bananas

Beets

Carrots

Peaches

Pumpkin

Sweet potatoes

FIRST FOODS EATEN FRESH

Avocado

Ripe banana

Peaches without skin and patted dry

Plums without skin and patted dry

Watermelon

Soft, very ripe melons

Roasted Sweet Potato and Banana

1 sweet potato
1 banana

1. Heat the oven to 350°F. Leave the sweet potato whole if it is small to medium or divide it in half if it is large. Wrap the sweet potato and banana (leaving the skins on) separately in foil.
2. Roast the sweet potato for one hour. During the last 20 minutes, roast the banana. Remove the banana and sweet potato and let cool slightly.
3. Discard the skins. Mash the sweet potato and banana with a fork or puree in a blender or mini food processor. Leftovers can be refrigerated or frozen for later use.

Schedule and Volume of Feeding

Families want to know how often they should feed baby solid foods, and how much to serve. Know that there is no "one size fits all" answer to this question. In the first few months of feeding solid foods, you're not trying to replace formula or breast milk, but adding the experience of tasting and swallowing new foods. You still want your baby to continue to get the vast majority of calories and nutrients from breast milk or formula. Therefore, it makes most sense to time the introduction of solid foods after milk feedings or between milk feedings, and to stick with small bites.

If you're giving your baby food that is store-bought, know that a whole large jar is probably too much for a brand-new eater to take at a single meal. Start with one feeding a day, but as your baby develops a liking for solid food, you may find yourself quickly moving to two and three feedings a day, timed with family meals. In the next chapter, we will discuss in detail the importance of establishing a feeding schedule for your older baby. In these introductory weeks, the actual nutrition offered by solid foods is limited, so ease into a schedule that feels comfortable for you and your baby.

Dr. Yum's Tip: Skip the Juice!
Many families ask when they can begin introducing juice. We recommend that parents skip giving juice altogether. Store-bought juice (even 100 percent juice) is a processed food that introduces a surge of unnecessary calories and sugar to a child's diet without offering fiber to help release that sugar slowly. When we give kids juice, we are training them to crave sugar instead of appreciating the natural sweetness and flavors of real food. Plus, regular consumption of juice predisposes children to excess weight gain and tooth decay. When it comes to introducing the cup to your baby (discussed in detail in the next chapter), skip the juice. Once the cup is established, teach your baby to drink plain water instead.

WHAT ABOUT FOOD ALLERGIES?

For years, parents were advised to introduce one food at a time, allowing a few days to elapse between new exposures to help reveal any food allergies a baby may have. Also, parents were told to wait two to three years before introducing high-risk foods like peanuts, eggs, and fish. However, in a 2008 report, the American Academy of Pediatrics concluded that solid foods should not be introduced until four to six months and there is no strong evidence that waiting beyond this time frame protects against food allergies. Their report included commonly allergenic foods, like fish, eggs, and foods with peanut protein.[32] Based on this information, many pediatricians now advise that for babies without a history of eczema or a strong family history of food allergies, most whole foods can be introduced safely without the need to follow a particular schedule.

ETHAN'S STORY:
Learning to Love Solid Foods

At the Doctor Yum Project's kitchen, we teach a preschool food adventure class. Preschoolers attend with a parent, and we introduce simple nutrition concepts, cooking basics, and other developmental skills while preparing a healthy snack. When I teach these classes, there is often a younger sibling who comes along for the ride. Often these siblings end up joining in and trying things their parents may not have imagined they could eat. In one particular session, a mom brought her preschool-aged daughter to our class with a seven-month-old baby brother, Ethan, perched in a carrier on her chest. This little guy was curious about all the sights, sounds, and smells around him and seemed to be taking it all in. His older sister was an eager learner and was excited to try some of the new foods.

On the second day, we were presenting a lesson on sugar snap peas and hummus, which we made from scratch with the kids. I was admiring the baby and told his mom how curious he seemed about the lessons. "Yes," his mom said. "We have been trying to get him interested in solid food, but he just doesn't seem to like it yet." She went on to describe how over the past few weeks she had been introducing different types of store-bought baby food and how he did not seem to like any of them and appeared perfectly happy just breast-feeding. I listened to the story and finally said, "Maybe he needs more flavor and would prefer homemade food. I wonder if he would like our hummus?"

The "summer hummus" we were making with chickpeas, tahini, lemon zest, and basil would be a big flavor difference compared to the bland and watered-down baby food he had been trying. "You really think he could try it?" his mom asked. "Just try a little finger-ful and see how it goes!" I said. "You never know until you try, right?" Much to this mom's surprise, her food-hating son licked the hummus off her finger with happy smacking noises and then went back to her finger for more!

I gave Mom more ideas for things she could try, like roasted carrots and zucchini. At the next preschool class, his mom reported that she and her son had tried some of the homemade food ideas and overnight he became the happiest, hungriest little solid food eater! Proof that babies in this age group can have an appetite for taste experiences that are more intense than we may first believe. This baby needed more flavor in his food (and probably more texture) and once he had it he was happy to eat!

5

NOW THE JOURNEY GETS INTERESTING
Nine to Fifteen Months

What happens in the life of a baby between nine and fifteen months is nothing short of miraculous. In six short months, your baby will go from a stationary individual babbling syllables like "ba-ba" to a fast-moving, sure-footed toddler who speaks several words and seems to understand everything! This explosion in development parallels the explosion of food experiences your baby can have, too.

In this same time frame, babies can go from eating relatively bland pureed foods to experiencing a variety of food tastes, textures, and temperatures from your own adult dinner plate. This chapter describes how to guide your baby through this Renaissance period and take advantage while they are open to new foods. Baby is also experiencing a boost in brainpower these days, directly impacting her ability to communicate. The journey over the next six months is packed with powerful experiences, so off we go!

GROSS MOTOR SKILL DEVELOPMENT

- Why a crawling baby is often a good eater, too!
- How the wrong high chair contributes to picky eating
- Parenting Proactively: The importance of early intervention

A CLOSER LOOK:
The Link Between Gross Motor Development and Eating

Previously content to clutch and mouth larger toys, babies now have the fine motor coordination to rake up small objects with their fingers. Eventually they will learn to use a pincer grasp where the thumb and forefinger pick up bite-sized morsels of food. Plus, baby will soon begin to try to spoon-feed himself—a messy but joyful process! Developing a pincer grasp and learning how to use a spoon, like all fine motor skills, are dependent on a child's corresponding gross motor development. It is important that babies are first able to sit without support and spend plenty of time crawling in order to develop the necessary strength and stability in their core and shoulder muscles. Think of it this way: If you have ever had a sore shoulder, it's very difficult to write, even though the pen is held in the hand. That's because the fine motor skill of handwriting is dependent on shoulder stability, which is dependent on core strength. Remember the lyrics to that old song "Dem Bones"? "The finger bone's connected to the hand bone / the hand bone's connected to the arm bone / the arm bone's connected to the shoulder bone." It's true! It's all connected, and the development of fine motor skills are always dependent on gross motor stability.

Between nine and fifteen months of age, babies learn to do amazing things! The most obvious achievement is increased development of gross motor skills. At nine months, some babies may be crawling, though many do not perform the traditional crawl (or creep). Instead they may scoot on their bottoms, roll from place to place, or be happy just where they are! Six months later, at fifteen months, most babies are walking, either on their own or holding onto an adult's hand or objects. This transition is a huge leap that changes everyone in the family's life, most importantly your baby's. What does this have to do with eating? A baby needs age-appropriate gross motor skills in order to learn the fine motor skills commonly known as "bite, chew, and swallow."

How to Guide Your Child: Gross Motor Skills

Baby wants to move! It starts with tummy time, progresses to rolling over and "commando-crawling," and before you know it, she's crawling, pulling to stand, cruising the furniture, and walking—all in the next six months! The more you can participate in gross motor play and floor time with your baby, the faster she'll be able to stabilize the muscles related to eating. Place toys just beyond your baby's reach to encourage baby to move forward. As she gets stronger, add low pillows, or even one of your legs for her to climb over. Never leave baby alone with anything on the floor that she could get trapped under or that might suffocate her, like a heavy blanket. You want to be there for safety reasons, but also to parent proactively, guiding your child through her next stage in gross motor development.

 If your nine-month-old baby is having difficulty sitting without support or bearing his own weight on his legs, consult with your pediatrician, who may refer your child to a pediatric physical therapist or occupational therapist for a gross motor assessment. Welcome those professionals with open arms, as they are your child's first coach for the earliest sports: crawling, cruising furniture, and walking!

One of the simplest ways to support your child's fine and gross motor development is to purchase a feeding chair that is designed to be a perfect fit for babies sitting up on their own and can be adjusted as they grow. As noted in chapter 4 (see page 51), children six months and older who are able to sit up on their own will be more comfortable and sit at the table longer if they can sit with their pelvis slightly tilted forward. This stabilizing position allows children to focus on biting, chewing, and swallowing. The stable trunk anchors the arms so that baby can more easily pick up finger foods and utensils and bring them to the mouth. We suggest purchasing a chair that offers this ideal positioning: Baby's knees and ankles are resting at a ninety-degree angle, just like when you sit in a bigger chair and put your feet on the ground. Beware of the plastic square booster seats that strap to dining room chairs or the cloth versions that hook onto the table top. They don't provide the support suggested here and cause the child's pelvis to tilt backward, especially if the dining chair also has a tilt in the seat. Instead, consider a high chair where the tray can be removed and then simply push the chair up to the dining table to ensure that your child has the support he needs to feel comfortable while seated for the entire meal.

Wondering what this has to do with eating? Try sitting on a stool, legs dangling, and slump your back. How easy is it for you to eat? Better yet, sit up nice and straight, with lovely posture, for your entire meal. Hard to do, isn't it? Adults prefer support but kids *need* support while eating. Improper positioning in the high chair contributes to picky eating because it's exhausting to eat that way. So, kids want to get down from the table sooner. Plus, it impacts kids' ability to operate their mouths and swallowing mechanisms effectively. Set them up for success by providing them with the support they need at that table.

MEGAN'S STORY:
Sitting Pretty with a New Feeding Position

Can you picture this? An adorable, curly-head moppet named Megan, a feisty ten-month-old, is seated in her fancy designer high chair. She's ready for her first session of feeding therapy and Coach Mel has arrived at her home to be a feeding detective. Her parents have called me in to answer this question: Why is it that Megan is unable to finish a few jars of puree?

As I settled in to observe, Megan's daddy lovingly began to feed Megan her favorite mush. There she was, tilted way, way back in the chair, in the same position she used as a six-month-old, when her parents first introduced homemade baby food on the tip of a coated spoon. The problem is, it's four months later and Megan is a very different kiddo! Out of habit, Megan's parents were still using the reclined position of the high chair.

So, there she was, essentially in a toddler-sized La-Z-Boy recliner, and at first, she looked as happy as my husband on Super Bowl Sunday. (I was tempted to hand her the TV remote!) As Megan's father proudly brought the bright pink spoon to her mouth, she eagerly shifted her position and tried to reach it—but this required doing "baby crunches" with each spoonful. She was throwing her shoulders forward, jutting out her chin, and engaging her abdominal muscles like she was in toddler gym class. Even her little toes lifted at the same time, often hooking under the tip of the high chair tray just to gain some stability for the rest of her body. Although Megan loved the yummy applesauce, she eventually fatigued and began to turn her head away. Her parents were interpreting this cue as "I'm full," when in fact, she was communicating, "Phew! I'm tired!"

Once your little one is sitting up on her own, it's time to end the La-Z-Boy days. Even a slightly reclined position discourages kids from learning to manage finger foods, develop a pincer grasp, and explore all the foods on a high chair tray. Megan's parents had kept her reclined not only out of habit but because her high chair, like many on the market, was too wide for her little hips and she seemed to swim in it. As noted in chapter 4, because many high chairs are meant to be used up to three years of age, parents may need to roll up a few towels into small bolsters that provide the hip and trunk support when first transitioning to the upright position.

Megan's dad and I grabbed all the kitchen towels, bolstered up the sides, and even put one rolled towel beneath the high chair cover directly in line with the small of her back so that she had the best support possible. Most importantly, we made sure that Megan could still be buckled in for safety. The following week, her parents reported that she was still enjoying the purees but happily exploring all the options on her tray, and staying in her high chair longer now that she wasn't having to do sit-ups while eating![34]

FINE MOTOR SKILL DEVELOPMENT

- Why finger foods can be tricky—but oh so important for development!
- Strategies to help your child learn to eat with a spoon
- How to use a fork and not lose an eye
- Parenting with Patience: Allowing your child time to learn

The pincer grasp is a fine motor skill that advances week to week and is fun to boost along during play and mealtimes! When small pieces of melting cereals were introduced to your child at about eight months of age, you may have noticed your baby raking the cereal into the palm of his hand before putting his tiny fist toward his lips, hoping that some would find the way into his mouth. At about nine months of age, your child will start to use his thumb and forefinger by pinching the side of the thumb against the finger, rather than using the tip.

PARENT PATIENTLY It's tempting just to hand your baby a pouch of baby food. He'll slurp it right down! There's nothing wrong with the occasional pouch for convenience, but parenting with patience means taking the extra steps, when you can, to hand your baby a spoon and wait. Give him the time to figure out how to use a utensil. Problem solving is a vital part of this journey and contributes directly to your child's brain development. Frustration is a different scenario than problem solving, so when you sense it may be too hard, make it a tad easier for him. Providing a bit of help is supportive, but jumping in and doing it for him stops the learning process in its tracks.

A mature pincer grasp occurs when the child can pick up the piece of cereal with his index fingertip and the tip of his thumb, pinch the cereal with just enough pressure to hold it still, and maneuver it into his mouth. In play, the same concept is applied to toys, as baby's hands strengthen over time. You may notice that your child uses his middle finger with his thumb. This will likely shift to a mature pincer grasp with time, as he becomes stronger and more coordinated.

Learning to use a spoon is another exciting milestone at this age! "Learning" is the key word here, as it's a messy process that takes time and has several steps. By nine to ten months of age, your baby has better control of simply dipping a spoon into a bowl and pulling it back out. It takes a bit more practice to get the "bowl" of the spoon into his mouth, and it's likely he'll flip the spoon over, spilling the contents right down his bib! That's because the first step to spoon-feeding is dipping, and learning to rotate the wrist so the spoon lands squarely on the tongue without spilling is a much more advanced step. Give your baby time to figure it all out. We don't expect kids to have mastered the spoon until fifteen months of age, and even then, we expect them to still be messy! At this stage, your toddler will also begin using a fork with relative ease, but mastery occurs around the age of two. Why is this important? If picking up morsels of food and learning to use utensils is challenging, toddlers may limit their food choices.

Coach Mel's Tip: Ready, Aim, Eat!
Using a permanent marker, color a wide stripe around the spoon handle so baby has a consistent spot to aim for when grabbing the spoon!

How to Guide Your Child: Fine Motor Skills

Throughout the day, there are lots of fun opportunities to build finger strength while practicing the pincer grasp. Take an old oatmeal box, cut a slit in the lid, and have fun dropping in metal baby food lids from those jars of baby food you no longer need! During bath time, use rubber bath toys that squirt when squeezed with two fingers. During mealtimes, hold a round piece of cereal in your own fingers, using a pincer grasp, and offer the cereal to your child. Hang onto it as he practices grabbing it with his thumb and forefinger.

Another fun activity is placing one piece of cereal in a plastic "shot glass" or similar-sized narrow container. The container should be approximately two inches tall and just wide enough for your child's thumb and forefinger to reach in and pull out the cereal. He'll have to use a pincer grasp to be successful. While you're at the coffee shop, entertain your child by stringing three pieces of circular cereal that melts in the mouth on a coffee stirrer. Hold it perpendicular to the tabletop and let your child pull off the cereal one by one using his thumb and forefinger.

You may be thinking this is a lot of effort just to teach finger-feeding! Actually, learning to use a pincer grasp in a controlled manner leads to future success in many other life skills: holding a pencil in preschool, fastening snaps, zippers, and buttons, and even cutting with scissors. You're helping your child with future achievements—and who knows, when he reaches out to grab that college diploma, you can say to yourself, "Glad I worked on that pincer grasp!"

Spoon-feeding is another fine motor skill that will develop with time. Dipping is the first step to learning to use a spoon; scooping food out of the bowl comes later. To help your baby learn to dip, don't hesitate to dip fingers first! Put just a smear of puree at the bottom of a bowl and dip your finger in it, bring it up to your mouth, and make a loud POP! Your baby will giggle with delight

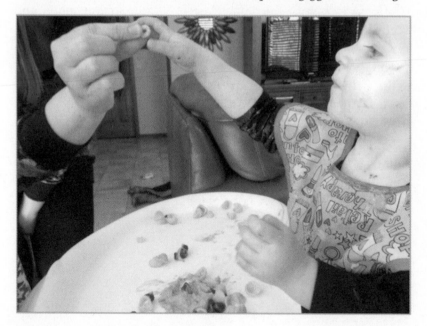

and try it, too! Once he's learned to dip a finger, give him a narrow chewie or a special spoon made just for dipping, like the NumNum dipper found at numnumdips.com.

If you're confident your child cannot bite off a chunk of it, a fat, peeled carrot makes a great dipper, too. Once baby is a master dipper, begin to teach the fine art of scooping. Be sure to choose the right spoon for little fists. A thick, short handle with a slight curve to it is ideal, so that baby naturally grabs the handle in just the right place. Too long of a handle will cause her to hold it toward the tip, and it's much too hard to maneuver the spoon into the mouth that way. The closer her tiny fist is to the bowl of the spoon, the more easily she will be able to guide the spoon into her mouth. A fun way for kids to practice spoon-feeding is to use the Baby Dipper Bowl found at babydipper.com. Invented by a mom of two sets of twins, the interior surface of the bowl slopes like a slide. Simply coat the slide with a small amount of puree. When baby dips the spoon into the bowl, she cannot help but dip and then scoop as the spoon travels down the slide. Plus, the spoon and the fork that come with the bowl are the perfect size for this developmental stage.

Learning to use a child-sized fork is the next fine motor skill. Choose a fork with the same type of handle as the spoon and with slightly rounded tines for safety. Be careful the fork is not too big for little mouths, as some child-sized forks are actually meant for kids over the age of three. When practicing fork-stabbing skills, use a plastic ice cube tray and place one cube of a soft food in each square. The sides of the "cubicle" act as a barrier, so the food can't roll away from the fork. Plus, the sides keep the fork contained too, so piercing the food is that much easier. We want kids to feel the success first, then graduate to more challenging fine motor tasks, like using a fork on a partitioned plate and eventually, on a flat plate just like his parents!

Be present with your child and use your powers of observation and intuition to understand what is working and not working as your child is feeding. Paying attention to what is going on in that little mouth will allow you to guide your child through these first stages of feeding successfully.

A CLOSER LOOK:
Thank Goodness for Proprioception!

Proprioception refers to our own awareness of where our various body parts are in space. Our brain considers how much strength or effort must be utilized to move each part in a coordinated and effective manner. Coach Mel's poor proprioception is why she constantly bangs her knee on the edge of her desk when she stands up too quickly, even though that desk has been in the same spot for the past ten years.

For children who are developing their sense of proprioception, learning to control a fork in order to stab a food like a cooked carrot can be tricky. Stab too hard and the carrot breaks into pieces or hold the fork at the wrong angle and the carrot becomes orange mush. As a child's muscles contract and stretch with each attempt at piercing the carrot, the brain receives proprioceptive input to communicate exactly what is happening and, thus, how to adjust and grade the movement in order to get the carrot on the tines of the fork. With practice and repeated input to the brain, eventually a child learns to stab the carrot and then fine-tune the movements so that the carrot ends up in the mouth and not up the nose.

CLOSER LOOK:
Important Changes in Oral Motor Development

The term "oral motor" refers to fine motor movements in the mouth, most often used for speech and eating—how we move our mouths in a coordinated and smooth fashion. As gross motor skills rapidly progress between the ages of nine to fifteen months, babies also make swift advancements in oral motor coordination, strength, and stability. Basically, they can move their mouths more and more like grown-ups, but they still have a way to go before biting into luscious tenderloin at the holiday dinner! Thanks to the bite reflex (discussed in chapter 3) integrating into the nervous system, babies start to gain control over how hard they bite down on food, grading their movements differently for a cracker versus a soft piece of potato. They'll need more practice on softer food before tackling chewy meats or food that doesn't dissolve

ORAL MOTOR SKILL DEVELOPMENT

- Why a sensitive gag reflex can stop a baby from trying new foods
- Does your child have an "immature" swallow pattern? It might lead to picky eating
- Is your toddler chewing, or just squishing the food?

By now, your baby's gag reflex has shifted from the front of the mouth to the back of the tongue. Your child has a new tolerance for tactile input in her mouth because she has been mouthing toys since birth. As your baby gains more control over holding toys and chews on them, this repeated tactile input signals her brain to be less troubled by the sensation, so she is less likely to gag when safe toys enter the mouth. Frequent exposure to new foods has also taught baby's brain to settle down. As baby learns to manage the new tastes, temperatures, and textures, the gag reflex is inhibited. Occasionally, you'll observe a loss of control when easily, like raw vegetables. The transverse tongue reflex pushes food onto the molars to be chewed and then retrieves the food so baby can swallow it. This movement is now becoming more controlled—baby is moving his tongue purposely to each side of his mouth!

Swallowing patterns are also changing. By twelve months of age, babies have almost mastered a mature swallow pattern, where the tongue tip elevates to the alveolar ridge (the bumpy spot where you make the "d" sound) just above the top teeth. No longer a forward-backward movement, a mature swallow begins with tongue tip elevation. Then, like magic, the edges of the tongue elevate to form a trough, holding the food until a muscular wave-like movement occurs from the tip to the back of the tongue, transporting the food toward the throat to be swallowed. A mature swallow is a clean swallow and very little food squirts to the side or through the lips, as previously observed in the six- to eight-month-old. Oral motor skills are pretty impressive at this age, aren't they?

the toy slips back and elicits a gag, but this is all part of the learning process. While the occasional gag may be tolerable, watch out for frequent gagging. This can lead to picky eating because kids begin to refuse new foods that may cause them to gag.

Tongue Thrusting and Teeth

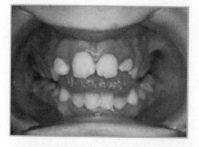

Don't let this photo of tongue thrusting scare you! The dentist has used a clear dental appliance to help you view the opening between the teeth, while the tongue is seen pushing through that space during the swallow.

Tongue thrusting can impact speech and feeding development as well as social aspects of eating. A child who thrusts the tongue may have difficulty controlling saliva, may be a messy eater, or suffer from digestive problems because of swallowing air throughout the meal.

Imagine how difficult it must be to keep food in the mouth and swallow effectively and efficiently! Notice the changes in this child's teeth—do you think he might have been a thumb sucker or had a pacifier in his mouth a lot? Possibly, and this tongue-thrusting pattern can persist into preschool and later years because now the tongue has a habit of moving forward and backward, rather than just resting in the mouth or lifting the tip when it comes time to swallow.

This pattern is just one of the aspects treated in the realm of "orofacial myofunctional disorders," where negative effects on dentition and facial development are addressed. A certified orofacial myologist can help your child change this pattern of swallowing.

How to Guide Your Child: Oral Motor Skills

You can help your baby learn to chew on the section of the gums where future molars will appear by placing small pieces of food directly on that area. By now, your baby should be comfortable with your fingers entering his mouth.

1. Cut soft, squishy foods, such as cooked carrots, baked potato, avocado, or soft cheeses into pea-sized cubes, and place them directly on the gums or molar area.
2. Gently push the cube on the molar area. Use firm pressure to ensure that his brain detects the food in that spot. When you press down, it provides the proprioceptive feedback (described in chapter 2) that tells your baby where the food is and directs the tongue to move toward that stimulation.
3. Your baby will bite down while his tongue moves laterally toward the piece of food. This downward motion, combined with the sideways movement of the tongue, will eventually develop into a rotary chewing pattern, which is how adults break up food during the chewing process.

Placing a pea-sized piece of food directly on the molar area increases the likelihood that the food will move to the back of the throat to be swallowed. When soft solids are placed on the tip of the tongue, and baby's forward-backward suckle pattern is still present, it is very likely the food will simply be pushed out of the mouth. Your baby's ability to transport the food from the tip of the tongue to the molar area for chewing is unlikely to be fully developed by nine months. When babies put food directly onto their tongues, they typically place it behind the tip, just squishing the food between the roof of their mouth and their tongue before swallowing it. Placing small portions directly on the gums encourages baby to practice the chew instead of the squish.

Coach Mel's Tip: Minimizing Baby's Gag Reflex

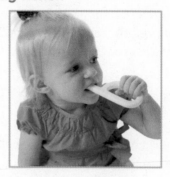

If you notice your baby gagging as he mouths new foods and toys, try not to give it too much attention because it's a natural part of learning, but watch to be sure that he is safe. To help shift the gag trigger to the back of the tongue, continue to offer a variety of safe foods and toys for baby to explore. Chewable toys may also help new teeth come in. Offer your baby long chewies, like the one from ARK Therapeutic pictured here, to shift the gag reflex toward the back of the tongue and to help your baby's chewing skills progress. Be sure that your child is mouthing and chewing those toys on the gums where future molars will soon erupt. If baby prefers to keep the tip of the toy near the front of his mouth, manipulate the toy and slowly move it toward the more sensitive areas, using firm yet gentle pressure. Playing with your child with teethers and chewable toys teaches the tongue a few tricks necessary for chewing and swallowing. Sing, smile, and make it fun!

But what about biting using the front teeth? That's still an important skill, and one that kids master slowly when mouthing and biting large soft pieces of food, like a wedge of ripe pear. Biting with the front teeth also includes moving the food from the tip of the tongue to the sides of the mouth to be chewed. In order to do so, your baby needs to develop strength and coordination on the sides of the tongue and throughout the jaw muscles. You can also use chew toys to develop this skill. As you or your baby manipulates the toy on baby's gums, the tongue will reach toward the toy in order to give the brain feedback about what is inside baby's mouth. That reflexive movement has now become more intentional as baby purposefully moves his tongue toward the toy to control the toy's movement with something other than his hands. The tongue begins to counterbalance the weight of the toy, becoming stronger in the process.

You're helping your baby practice how to manipulate food in his mouth, keep the food on his molars for chewing, and retrieve it when ready to swallow.

Cognitive Skills Related to Feeding

One of the primary cognitive skills that will begin to influence your child's behavior at mealtimes is her use and understanding of language. In the period of nine to eighteen months of age, children generally understand language better than they can express it. Research shows that teaching your baby sign language can boost verbal language development in these early years.[35] Baby's imitation skills are blossoming and it's amazing how many signs they learn to use! Plus, sign language keeps communication frustrations to a minimum and that's especially important at mealtimes. Now, she can request certain foods using sign and verbal language, and can express her preferences when a certain food is not to her liking.

You'll also observe your baby's "pretend play" emerging over time, especially when pretending to feed baby animals, dolls, and even superheroes! Child-size plates, cups, and utensils aren't just for use in the high chair. Be sure your child's play area is stocked with miniature pots, pans, and kitchen fare so that your little chef can cook and feed his playroom friends. Count the number of "steps" that your child performs in dramatic or pretend play. By eighteen months, some (but not all) children are demonstrating two-step pretend play with ease—for example, she might bottle-feed her stuffed bear and then burp him, then repeat. You'll notice that she is likely beginning to use two-word phrases, too. Three-step play would involve feeding the bear the bottle, burping him, and then putting him to bed. You can facilitate this cognitive development by practicing two-step play and mastering that, then introducing three-step play. Don't be surprised if your child picks up a stick and pretends to feed her favorite stuffed animal with it! Pretend play is also called "symbolic play" when kids use one object as a symbol for another, like a stick for a spoon. Her first words and/or signs are also symbols in the world of language, so it's important to help her develop symbolic play as a means of developing language.[36]

DRINKING WITH STRAWS, OPEN CUPS, AND SIPPY CUPS

- How straws and open cups encourage a child to try new tastes
- Sippy cups: Why we recommend just skipping them!

By nine months, most babies are ready to practice drinking from a cup. Bottle-fed babies can start practicing so that by their first birthday they are able to wean from the bottle. For babies who are breast-fed, try offering an open cup with water between nursing. Some breast-fed babies may start to wean naturally, and building skills to drink confidently from a cup means that they will be ready to progress when that happens.

A CLOSER LOOK:
Sippy Cups (and Why You May Not Need Them!)

Feeding therapists often observe that drinking liquids of thick consistency through a straw builds strength and stability in the lips, mouth, jaw, and tongue. Think about that last milkshake or smoothie you drank . . . did your mouth muscles get tired? If your child is in speech or feeding therapy, a "straw program" may be implemented, but why not also offer Greek yogurt or other thick foods via a straw at home? It's fun, and it just might help with speech and feeding development! The thicker the food and the thinner the straw, the harder those muscles have to work.

While a short straw assists in developing the mature swallow pattern, a spouted sippy cup does not. Sippy cups became all the rage in the 1980s, along with oversized shoulder pads, MC Hammer parachute pants, and bangs that stood up like a waterspout on top of your head. A mechanical engineer, tired of his toddler's trail of juice throughout the house, successfully designed a spill-proof cup and Playtex licensed the product. The rest is history. Today, a generation of parents appears to believe that transitioning from breast or bottle to the sippy cup is part of the developmental process of eating. But it's not: Using a sippy cup has little to do with learning to drink or eat.

The issue is that those sippy cups seem to linger through preschool. Speech-language pathologists and dentists have observed that prolonged use can to lead to incorrect tongue posture (how we use and rest our tongues in our mouths), and the hard spout held in the mouth over time may impact dentition, palate formation, and facial features. While research is needed to determine how long a child should use a spouted sippy cup, you may decide to limit them to occasional use over a few months. Or, now that your child drinks from a short straw, you may step away from them altogether. With so many pop-up straw cups on the market that limit spills, it's possible!

Coach Mel's Tip: Children with Special Needs May Benefit from Sippy Cups
For kids with special needs, a specialist in swallowing disorders may recommend a spouted or sippy cup due to concerns of aspiration (breathing in liquid). Please follow the recommendations of your child's medical professional first and foremost.

How to Guide Your Child: Straws and Open Cups

Straws

You can begin to cultivate a mature swallowing pattern, where the tip of the tongue elevates to the alveolar ridge (remember, that's where you put your tongue to say the "d" sound), by teaching your nine-month-old how to drink from a straw. This teaches the tongue to lift up and then creates a controlled wave that slides the food back to be swallowed. Before starting, your baby must first be accepting a spoon filled with smooth puree with ease, cleaning off the spoon using her upper lip, and eating at least three ounces of pureed baby food in this manner without fatiguing. Straw drinking offers quite the workout for mouth muscles and is a more advanced oral motor skill!

When teaching drinking through a straw, always start with a smooth puree, not a thin liquid, which is actually too difficult for babies to manage at first because it spreads too quickly across the tongue. Limit the amount in the straw to two to three inches of puree so as not to startle your child who is experiencing the sensation for the very first time.

To teach your child to drink from a straw, follow these ten easy steps:

1. Open a full jar of your child's favorite smooth, pureed baby food. Either homemade or store-bought is fine.
2. Dip a short, firm-sided straw in the puree, then let the tip fill about ½-inch full, so that there is puree inside and outside the straw. Put your finger on top of the straw to prevent the puree from spilling out the bottom.

3. With your finger still on the top of the straw, place about ½ inch of the wet straw flat on your child's tongue, as if it were a spoon of puree.

4. Wait for your child's lips to close around the puree on the tip, let go of the top hole, and slowly draw the straw straight out of his mouth. The tiny bit of puree that was on the outside of the straw is now on your child's tongue, ready to be swallowed.

5. Continue with this process until your child can manage a tiny bit more puree inside the straw. Remember, the outside of the straw should have a little puree on it, too, to tempt his lips to close around it.

6. Once your child has mastered steps 1 through 5 (this can take a few days of practice or happen all in one day), prime the straw with the puree two to three inches from the bottom by sucking on the top of the straw and then putting your finger over the top hole. Be sure to dip the bottom of the straw in just a tiny bit of puree, so that when you present it again, your child feels the puree on the outside.

7. To teach the next step, the suck, the key is to leave the straw in your child's mouth one to two seconds longer. Present the straw just as you would a spoon, wait for her lips to close . . . now wait again. As soon as she begins to suck, lift your finger off the top hole so that the puree can flow. Let your child suck slowly and swallow repeatedly until the straw is empty.

8. Once your child can manage two inches with ease, prime the straw to the top (four to five inches). Let your child practice sucking all the puree through the straw, as described in step 7.

9. Take the full jar of food (or a covered cup filled to the top with puree) and leave about one inch of straw tip sticking out above the puree. Add a dab of puree to the tip of the straw again, just to encourage the sucking action. You may need to hold the jar or cup at a 45-degree angle so that the straw enters his mouth at just the right position while he learns to suck and prime the straw on his own.

10. Now that your child has mastered drinking purees via a straw, gradually thin the puree with water to nectar consistency and, eventually, to just plain water. Congratulations! Your child can now drink any consistency through a straw!

Once your child can drink this way, it's time to cut the straw short enough that it extends just past the lips and barely touches the tip of the tongue resting in the mouth. Why? If the straw is too long, the tongue tip cannot lift to swallow properly.

 Coach Mel's Tip: Use a Silicone Straw
For younger, more sensitive mouths, bendable yet sturdy silicone straws can be purchased from the popular speech and feeding therapy website talktools.com.

Open Cups

Open cups are typically introduced before the age of one, when baby is reaching for your glass and wants to see what's inside! The larger "mouths" of an adult cup are too big for babies. They can't make a tight enough seal on them with the corners of their lips. (Imagine how you would feel learning to drink from a bucket!) When holding a cup of liquid for baby, offer it in a small container, such as a tiny baby food jar, small juice glass, or even a shot glass. The rims are just the right size for little mouths, and since you will be the one to hang on to the container, the clear glass makes it easier for you to see baby's mouth. In the next chapter, we'll discuss how to teach independent open-cup drinking, even with a glass container.

The right cup and straw can encourage kids to explore new tastes. Thinner straws allow just a tiny amount of a liquid to land on the tongue. By sucking on a straw, your child gets a quick taste and then a swallow. Thin straws are perfect (and fun!) tools for introducing soups, sauces, or nut-based milks. Slightly wider straws provide a bit more liquid on the tongue, and thus, a bit more taste. Using the widest straws, like those for thicker drinks like smoothies, really packs a punch of flavor!

If your child is sensitive to smells, a cup with a lid and a straw can help her explore new tastes without being turned off by an aroma. Open cups, especially small ones easily held in little fists, enable the most interaction with new foods, even purees. Their little noses are deep in the cup, and lips, tongue, and teeth are all experiencing the delicious food you've poured for them. Try these cups with liquids or thinned-down mashed turnips, mashed potatoes, or smoothies. The thicker purees will prove to be easier to manage than thin liquids when children are first learning to use an open cup.

LETTING GO OF THE PACIFIER OR THUMB

- Don't let these contribute to picky eating!
- Parenting Bravely: Weaning your child from the pacifier and thumb

As discussed in chapter 4, the nonnutritive suck instinct is nature's way of helping a baby calm himself. But by three months of age, your baby has gained some control over the reflex to suck and may turn away when you place your finger in his mouth. Between nine and twelve months of age, a child no longer needs a pacifier or thumb, unless the child has a highly sensitive sensory system (see chapter 2). This is partly because of the conditioned response of sucking paired with other soothing behaviors, such as being held in Mom or Dad's arms before bedtime or the soft feel of a favorite "lovey" as baby falls asleep. The paired stimulus—the hug or the lovey—is now what calms the child and the sucking behavior fades away. Plus, because children are programmed to explore the world with their hands, fingers, and mouths, and you have provided baby with age-appropriate chew toys and foods, your child is getting the important oral input for mouth development via play and eating. How is this related to picky eating? Well, it's hard to explore the world of food when a thumb or pacifier is in the way! Plus, anything resting on the tongue prevents the tip from elevating for that important mature swallow pattern to develop.

CLOSER LOOK:
Pacifiers

Typically, a child develops the mature swallow pattern needed for managing more challenging foods between nine and fifteen months. Prolonged use of the pacifier or thumb prevents the tongue tip from lifting up and propelling the saliva backward to be swallowed, because the paci is in the way. Instead, the tongue pushes forward, under the pacifier. While we need studies to determine what "prolonged use" means, research shows that pacifier use past the age of two contributes to poor teeth alignment and changes in bone formation in the mouth.[37] Consider letting go of the pacifier during the day by baby's first birthday, and limit it to bedtime use up to the age of eighteen months. Saying goodbye to the pacifier is much easier for a one-year-old than an older toddler because he has not become as dependent on it.

A recent publication showed that in just one year in the United States there were more than 42,000 injuries from bottles, pacifiers, and sippy cups. The majority of injuries were to one-year-olds and included lacerations and lost and broken teeth.[38] This is not difficult to imagine because this is an age when babies are starting to walk, are unsteady on their feet, and fall frequently.

Dr. Yum's Tip: Preventing Injuries

Limit the pacifier to the crib, when your child is resting. For additional safety, try to keep kids seated while drinking from bottles or cups.

How to Guide Your Child: Getting Rid of Pacifiers and Thumb-Sucking Behavior

Pacifiers

The first step is to limit the pacifier to bedtime by six months of age. Whether you co-sleep or baby has his own crib, teach your child that you will gently take the pacifier out of the mouth and place it on the mattress *before* you lift baby out of bed. Here are three methods that parents find easier on them and their child, regardless of the age that parents decide to "let go" of the pacifier:

1. WubbaNub pacifiers come attached to small stuffed animals, thus pairing the comfort of sucking with stroking a "lovey." Gather *all* the WubbaNubs in the house and cut off the pacifiers on every animal but one. Discard all the pacifiers. When you're ready, do the same for the last pacifier. We recommend doing this on garbage pickup day, so you aren't tempted to retrieve them from the trash in a moment of desperation. Now, your child has a lovey to soothe him while sleeping. Ideally, keep the lovey in the crib, so that your child doesn't become dependent on needing it away from bedtime.

2. Build-a-Bear Workshops are in most shopping malls across the country, where kids of all ages create their own stuffed animals from start to finish, including stuffing them to the "just right" amount of fluff. Once again, gather all the pacifiers in your home and discard all but one. Bring your child to Build-a-Bear, explaining that it's time to get a special friend to help him fall asleep. When it comes time to stuff the bear, the attendant at the workshop will place the pacifier in the bear's ear (or preferred spot), fill the bear with stuffing, and sew the bear shut. Now, your child can still feel the pacifier, reassured that it's there, and has an extra soft friend to cuddle with at night. Parents, you are not allowed to cut open that bear! Parent bravely!

3. The "it's broken, can't fix it" method takes a bit of time, but is very inexpensive to implement and is most successful with kids eighteen months and up. Begin by leaving a few broken items around the house, such as a pencil broken in half on the kitchen counter. Pick it up and show it to your toddler, saying, "Oh, it's broken, can't fix it," and throw it in the trash. After a week of introducing this concept, take the pacifier that is in the crib and snip off the tip when your child is not there. Discard the tip. Put your child to bed a bit early that day, so that she isn't too tired to encounter the broken pacifier. This is a bittersweet moment to capture on video, because your little one will likely hold up the pacifier and say, "Bwoken." Give her a big hug and take her and the pacifier to the trash can to throw it away. Then, put your child in her crib again and pour yourself a glass of wine . . . consider it doctor's orders. Seriously, you and your child will be fine without the pacifier. Give yourself three days to get through the final good-byes and then celebrate how brave you both were!

 Saying good-bye to the paci is often harder on the parents! We understand—the pacifier is such a relief to have on hand! Remember to parent bravely: You were armed with the knowledge of why your child may have benefited from a pacifier and now you're also aware of why it's important to wean her at an early age. Knowing this can make weaning the pacifier easier when the time comes.

Thumb Sucking

Breaking the thumb-sucking habit is naturally more challenging, because the thumb is always there. We've listed three strategies that may be a good fit for you and your child, but if the habit persists into the preschool years, consult with a certified orofacial myologist (OFM) who is trained in breaking the sucking habit. Your pediatric dentist can refer you to an OFM in your area, or you can visit the International Association of Orofacial Myology at iaom.com for a list of certified practitioners. Another excellent resource is the book *How to Stop Thumb Sucking* by Pamela Marshalla, MA, CCC-SLP. In her book, Marshalla notes that the young toddler years are the ideal time to begin weaning from the thumb. She reports that toddlers' behaviors are changing rapidly at this time, and they can be encouraged to sample other means of oral play and other things to do with their hands, thanks to their need to explore.[39]

Here are some tips that can help your toddler gently give up thumb sucking:

1. From the age of six months, whenever your child puts his thumb in his mouth, give him something to chew and suck on instead. Begin to shape the change in the behavior.

2. Offer alternatives for calming that don't involve thumb sucking when your child is young, such as infant massage, rocking while holding a large stuffed animal, or swaddling. As children grow, the more opportunities they have to self-calm in a variety of ways, the less dependent they will be on the thumb.

3. The more your child has the chance to engage in safe fine motor skill activity, the better! Busy fingers rarely find their way into the mouth and you'll be improving your child's dexterity, too.

 Coach Mel's Tip: Give Your Child a "Chewie" Be sure to offer age-appropriate chewies throughout the day to provide the calming oral input that kids need, especially when giving up the pacifier or thumb. Some of our favorites are the adorable breakaway safety necklaces, clip-ons on organic lanyards, and soft "chewelry" by kidcompanions.com.

PROGRESSING THROUGH SOLID FOODS

- Why variety truly is the spice of life—even for your baby!
- Finger foods: Looking beyond cereal that melts in the mouth

As you're learning, there is a ton of development that happens in these six short months! There is a lot of variability in the pace of babies' motor skill development, and one baby can progress faster in certain areas than the next. Similarly, the pace in which solid foods can be comfortably introduced may be different from one baby to another. But in general, a child's skills are increasing quickly during this time, and so can the tastes and textures of the foods you present. And you have opportunities to stave off picky eating! Research shows that parents who wait to offer a variety of "lumpy" food until babies are ten months or older are more likely to have "fussy eaters" by the age of fifteen months, and those children are more likely to prefer purees even after age one.[40]

How to Guide Your Child: Good-bye Purees, Hello Real Food!

So here's the fun part! As your child progresses through this period, your family can involve baby in mealtime by serving foods similar to what the rest of the family is eating, including stews, casseroles, pasta, soft meats, and more. Now is the time to limit the melt-in-your-mouth rice puffs (your baby will grow tired of them quickly, anyway!) and consider a few of these more "grown-up" options. At nine months, babies are now ready for lots of new tastes, textures, and experiences. Once you get going, you will be surprised at how quickly feeding can advance. Babies are ready, open, and *hungry* for new foods. They are still in a period of rapid growth at this age and being hungry is the direct result!

With this surge in hunger, you might be wondering how much food to put on baby's high chair tray. Our answer is: just enough to entice, but not so much as to overwhelm. For a nine-month-old, starter portions at mealtimes may include two tablespoons of a protein, half slice of toast with smeared avocado, and two table-spoons of a chopped soft fruit or vegetable. Then, offer more according to baby's appetite. For fifteen-month-olds, offer slightly more, perhaps three tablespoons. Your child can certainly have more at mealtimes, but offering small portions at first peaks baby's interest and lets him tune in to the feelings of hunger. Watching your baby's communication cues is more important that having a chart of how much to feed. Signs that baby is full or disinterested in eating include turning away, beginning to be more focused on playing with the food than putting it in his mouth, and eating slower with more time between bites. Being in touch with these cues will help teach your baby how to listen to his own signs of fullness and eat just the amount that his body needs.

Foods to Keep Your Baby on the Road to Adventurous Eating

Here are some foods that your new eater can explore while you include him in your family's eating experience and food culture.

Stews: Cook lots of different ingredients into a big stew that can feed the whole family. Add sweet potatoes, carrots, greens, and beans, and don't be afraid to throw in slices of apple or squash to add other nutrients. Also, be sure to include herbs and seasonings to keep the taste buds guessing. You can serve a stew alone in a bowl or over rice, as shown in the Lentils with Spinach recipe at the end of this chapter. Early on, take a ladleful of stew and give it a whirl in the blender. As babies get used to more texture, you will need to blend less. Making the stew thick will allow babies who are learning to self-feed spoon it to their mouths with more success. Plus, the beauty of a stew is that you can save samples of each vegetable for the "sides," so that kids discover each food individually and as a mixed dish.

Dairy products: Cow's milk as a primary food source is generally not advised before one year, as it tends to be low in iron. However, small amounts of cheese are OK in this phase and can be one of the soft foods that are easy to introduce. For a dose of immune-building probiotics, introduce yogurt. Just make sure that the yogurt you choose is not too heavily sweetened. You may be surprised to discover that even brands geared toward babies can be very high in sugar.

Fruits and veggies: Steamed or roasted veggies and soft, ripe fruits make for great finger foods. Dice them into small pieces, or even better, into thin strips that can be held easily and break off when placed in the mouth.

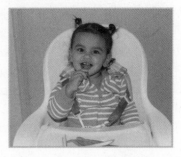

Pasta: Make soft pasta and stir it with sauces that include fresh vegetables in bite-size pieces. Don't be afraid of rich sauces. Babies at this age still need fat for brain growth and development. Bow-ties may be too big for those kids brand-new to finger foods, so start with a smaller, more manageable shape, like elbow macaroni.

Bread: Toast whole grain bread and cut it into bite-size pieces. Many parents are surprised to hear that lightly toasted bread is easier for young children to manage than bread that is not toasted. Spread it with hummus, which is high in protein and can introduce new flavors. Sweeter breads and muffins have a moist, soft texture and can be torn into easy-to-chew bites. When made at home, they can also be prepared with healthy whole grains or gluten-free, and can include many nutritious ingredients, like small pieces of baked apple.

Coach Mel's Tip: Toast That Bread!
It's easier for your baby's mouth to feel toast than un-toasted bread. Be sure to butter it generously, or add a nutritious, oily spread like smashed avocado, to help bind the pieces while they are chewed and moisten them for swallowing.

Meatballs: Ground meat is a great way to introduce a protein with a soft and moist texture. Incorporate spices and finely shredded veggies with your favorite ground meat to make flavorful meatballs with added nutrients. At first, make mini-meatballs (or meat-bites!) just a centimeter in size. Alternately, make giant meatballs so kids can learn to bite off easy-to-swallow bites. Meatballs can be made softer and more flavorful by adding them to soups. Don't hesitate to let kids scoop the meatballs out of the broth with spoons, stab with a fork, or even use their fingers. Add a straw to let baby sip the yummy broth.

 Dr. Yum's Tip: Try Whole Grains
Offer whole grains when possible. Brown rice, whole wheat pasta, and whole grain breads have a more complex taste and offer more nutrients and fiber than the refined white versions.

The Importance of a Feeding Schedule

With newborns, many parents feed on demand, offering the breast or bottle when their babies seem hungry. This strategy works for many reasons. For the breast-feeding mother, milk production is slow in the early days. Stimulating the breast often by feeding on demand can help her milk come in quickly. Also, newborns may need a more constant supply of calories to keep blood sugar in the normal range. However, as babies get older, developing an eating schedule that has strategic breaks can really help make their food journey successful. Not only does it create a predictable hunger cycle, it sets up mealtimes as devoted "eating times" when children can truly enjoy and experience food. This allows for "growing times," which are breaks from eating, when they can rest and work on other areas of development, like gross motor skills.

Experiencing and managing hunger is important for establishing healthy eating habits, and you can start this lesson by putting your baby on a feeding schedule. As parents, our instinct is to minimize hunger so children don't experience the sensation. But this can backfire. Many kids graze on food throughout the day, and then, when faced with the nutrient-packed meals their parents have prepared, their interest in eating falls flat. Whereas breast-feeding may be on demand, establishing a feeding schedule for breast-feeding also eases your baby into a new feeding schedule for solids. Successful parenting sometimes means presenting all types of experiences and giving kids the tools to manage them. Hunger is no exception.

 Creating a consistent feeding schedule allows kids to experience a hunger cycle, which may drive an interest in nutritious food at mealtimes. Grazing constantly throughout the day is an *inconsistent* response to feelings that are often not related to hunger. Instead, your child may be snacking in response to fatigue, thirst, emotions, or boredom with food.

How to Guide Your Child: Establishing a Feeding Schedule

Feeling hungry teaches kids to pay attention to all the sensations in their bodies and respond appropriately. By paying attention to hunger and responding by filling little bellies, you can help your kids grow up to become adults who eat in reaction to hunger, rather than eating in response to other feelings, like sadness, boredom, or anxiety.

Here is an example of a schedule that may work for babies of this age. Please note that "Eating Time" refers to the window of time in which you will sit down with your child for snacks or mealtimes. Children ages nine to fifteen months typically spend twenty minutes enjoying a meal and ten minutes for a snack. But if you're having a great time together and decide to sit longer to eat, just remember that the time span between meals and snacks, or "Growing Time," is two to two and a half hours. Afternoons may vary slightly as nap times can stretch out the time just a bit.

• •

MORNING: Breakfast Eating Time
Growing Time of 2 to 2½ Hours

MIDMORNING: Snack Eating Time
Growing Time of 2 to 2½ Hours

MIDDAY: Lunch Eating Time
Growing Time of 2 to 2½ Hours

MIDAFTERNOON: Snack Eating Time
Growing Time of 2 to 2½ Hours

EVENING: Dinner Eating Time

Notice the flexibility in the schedule. Ideally, kids do best when their daily routine is predictable. However, on some days you may get up later, so breakfast may be served later. This may lead to shifting the time you enjoy your midmorning snack. The ranges of eating times allow you to be responsive to your babies needs on a particular day. Also, notice the periods of time away from eating where other developmental skills can be explored, rest can happen, and hunger can develop. When babies are fussy, we sometimes misinterpret that as hunger and have a tendency to want to try feeding. After establishing a schedule where babies are used to eating or not eating at set times, it may be easier to take hunger out of the equation and avoid overfeeding. For example, you might say to yourself, "Maybe this fussiness is teething, and not hunger, since I just fed him his snack thirty minutes ago, and this usually satisfies him until lunchtime."

Dr. Yum's Tip: Patience!
Feeling hunger teaches kids the important skill of *waiting*!

Children's eating patterns will also shift in terms of what foods they will be interested in. At nine months, babies are still getting most of their calories and nutrients from milk, so some of the "snacks" will be a bottle of formula or breast milk. By fifteen months, much of a baby's nutrition comes from solid food, which will replace the snack-time bottle or some time breast-feeding. In general, when you and your baby become comfortable with these periods of eating and not eating, you're laying the groundwork for successful and adventurous eating for the long haul. At this stage babies are primed to try anything, but this wonderful phase may not last. As children get a little older, and at times more selective, having a schedule that allows for mild hunger will help them try new foods and emerge from those selective phases more easily. As the old saying goes, "Hunger is the best sauce."

By this age, your child has new teeth that are erupting. It is important to take care of these teeth by brushing twice a day with a soft toothbrush and a smear of toothpaste. It turns out that the changes in mouth pH that occur with eating can lead to tooth decay. When we eat, the pH in our mouths decreases to a level that can actually promote demineralization and decay. Taking breaks from eating allows the mouth pH to increase to a more neutral level, which helps restore teeth and keep them healthy.

HAVING FUN WITH FOOD!

- Why being messy is important
- How food exploration leads to eating more variety

Eating with Hands

Children are programmed to explore the world with their hands, fingers, and mouths. Although it may feel helpful to swipe a child's face with the spoon, wiping and swiping actually prevents kids from experiencing all the tactile aspects of food. Let kids handle the food themselves and just wipe messy hands and fingers with a wet rag, or cover kids in "super-bibs" that envelop everything from the tip of the chin to the edge of the wrists. As noted in chapter 2, where we discuss sensory integration, the more a child can learn about a new food with all of their senses, the more information they can store in their brain about different tastes, temperatures, and textures. That's how we all make decisions in life about what is safe, what is enjoyable, and what interests us. We compare it to prior information and decide if and how we want to proceed to interact with a similar experience—or similar food.

How to Guide Your Child: The Importance of Getting Messy

You may be thinking, "I want him to *stop* playing with his food and just *eat it*!" Keep in mind that for many kids, playing in their food leads to eating. But if you sense that too much messy play is instead distracting your child from eating, then keep the "playing" in food to play time, where you make pudding pictures and stack vegetable blocks. Get creative and incorporate food into other aspects of the day. Meanwhile, if your child is kept on a schedule for meals, hunger will override the tendency to play during mealtimes. Still, embrace the mess that naturally coincides with self-feeding, because at that very messy moment, your child is actively learning about food!

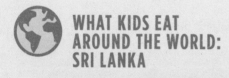

WHAT KIDS EAT AROUND THE WORLD: SRI LANKA

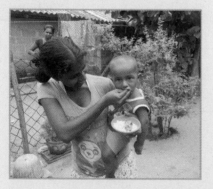

The island nation of Sri Lanka is a beautiful country in the Indian Ocean, with population that has a healthy diet and traditionally long life span. Generally, babies get their start eating solids around six months with native red rice, which is high in nutrients and fiber. Families cook the rice until very soft and feed babies by hand, smashing it as they go. By nine months, parents introduce other nutrients in a traditional "white curry." This is a mild blend of coconut milk, curry powder, and turmeric, which forms the base of the curry and allows the introduction of leafy greens and other soft vegetables, cooked together with the rice all in one pot.

Babies are offered the same meals as the rest of the family and fed on a similar schedule. Traditionally, meals like rice and curries are eaten with fingers and parents do their best to smash these soft foods, but often they are left a bit lumpy. Babies are also fed smashed bananas and other tropical fruit like mango. By one year, curry and more spices are introduced into the diet, along with other proteins like fish, lentils, and chicken. A particularly spicy dish with chili powder may be made milder with a white curry broth to dilute the heat. This early exposure to so many tastes and textures guarantees Sri Lankan children will adopt their native diet easily and with relatively little fuss.

When feeding their babies, Sri Lankans encourage their children to open their mouths *wide*. Like a long chewie or teether, the fingers stimulate the back of the child's mouth, helping to decrease the gag reflex and consequently helping feeding skills advance.

Lentils and Spinach over Rice

Traditional Sri Lankan dishes include lentils and spinach. Red lentils (which are pumpkin-colored) cook really quickly and can be mixed with rice into tiny rice balls, just right for little fingers to hold and enjoy! This is a complete meal with protein, grain, and leafy greens in one nutritious bite.

Serves 4 adults with leftovers for baby

1 tablespoon olive oil
1 onion, diced
2 cloves garlic, minced or pressed
1 small tomato, diced
1 teaspoon curry powder
¼ teaspoon turmeric
Chili powder to taste
1 cup red lentils, rinsed with cold water
2 cups baby spinach, finely chopped
⅔ cup coconut milk
Salt and pepper
2 to 3 cups cooked brown rice

1. Heat the olive oil in a medium saucepan. Cook the onions until soft, about 3 to 4 minutes. Then add the garlic and cook another 1 to 2 minutes. Cook the tomato for 2 minutes, or until soft. Mix in the curry powder, turmeric, and chili powder.

2. Add the lentils and enough water to cover them by ½ inch. Cook for 5 to 8 minutes, or until the lentils are soft. Add the spinach and coconut milk and simmer another 1 to 2 minutes, until spinach is wilted. Season with salt and pepper. Serve over brown rice.

TIP: Brown jasmine rice works well in this recipe, but experiment with other whole grain rice varieties, too. Make sure to cook with plenty of water so the rice is soft and easy to smash.

Variation:
Rice Balls with Lentils and Spinach for Babies

Take about one cup cooked brown rice. Add a teaspoon of the lentil-spinach mixture and mix by hand. Add more lentils by the teaspoon and keep mashing until you can form the mixture into ¾-inch balls.

Here's how to explain to relatives why your child needs to get messy. "It might look messy, but being able to explore food with all of her senses helps my child understand all the aspects of taste, temperature, texture, and more! If the messiness begins to be too distracting, we'll redirect her. But for now, she's learning about the joy of food! She's *experiencing* it—that's the key to becoming an adventurous eater. I'm excited that today she's smooshing butternut squash because someday she'll be ordering it off the fanciest menu!"

It's been an interesting trek thus far: The period from nine to fifteen months is a fast-paced leg of the journey, with a ton of learning and growing. Keep up with your baby's natural tempo when it comes to the food adventures and experiences you offer. Let her get messy, experience a wide variety of tastes and textures, and most importantly have fun while exploring new foods. Take it all in; it's just the beginning. You and your baby are setting the tone for an exciting and successful road ahead!

6

A BUMP IN THE ROAD
Sixteen to Twenty-four Months

These months can be a challenging time, even before the classic "terrible twos" start to emerge. It can be difficult to communicate with your toddler, as he still has limited language skills plus limitless demands. This disconnect can lead to you both feeling easily frustrated. Toddlers may also be unpredictable when it comes to their food preferences and appetite. However, know that at this stage your child has gained an incredible toolbox of gross and fine motor skills that will allow him to actively participate in the kitchen. You now have a tiny sous chef at your side! Engaging a child in kitchen activities can be a way to build their developmental skills and keep them familiar with, healthy whole foods, even if they don't always choose to eat them.

GROSS MOTOR SKILL DEVELOPMENT

- How running, jumping, and exploring leads to exploring food, too
- Parenting Proactively: Scheduling time to grow
- Parenting with Consistency: Setting boundaries

Your child is walking and is on the move! It's tricky to keep an eye on her while she gets into everything: opening cabinets, climbing over furniture, and negotiating obstacles. Your child is developing bilateral coordination skills, where she learns to move her right arm with her left leg (and vice versa) as she runs around the living room. She's also learning to move both legs together as she jumps from the ottoman to the carpet. Because she's on the move, she may not want to sit still to eat for very long and mealtimes can become a battle. This age can be frustrating, because not only are kids more active, but they can seem inconsistent in their appetite, moods, and food preferences. It's an opportunity to practice parenting with consistency, where you offer safe choices for gross motor skill development and healthy choices at mealtime.

 Understanding that kids' preferences may wax and wane doesn't change your style of parenting. Parenting with consistency requires us to set the boundaries around healthy choices while occasionally offering treats.

How to Guide Your Child: Gross Motor Skills

The best way to guide your child during this active phase is to provide just that: activity! Pull the cushions off the couch and move the ottoman to the center of the room. Create obstacle courses: mountains to climb and hills to roll down. Notice how your child uses both sides of his body: Is it coordinated? Is it smooth?

Bilateral coordination involves using both the left and right sides of the body for one action, like throwing a pillow straight up in the air. Or, it can involve alternating, coordinated movements, such as running around the living room. Bilateral coordination can also involve one side leading and the other side assisting in a task, such as holding on to the arm of the couch while lifting the opposite leg onto the couch cushion.

How does bilateral coordination help with mealtime behavior? By providing your child with practice using both sides of his body, you're establishing skills that enable him to hold a plate steady with one hand and scoop pinto beans with a spoon in the other. He'll be able to bite a burrito held in one hand, while reaching for milk in a cup. One day he'll be able to pick up a serving platter with both hands and carefully pass it around the Thanksgiving table. Eventually, he'll be ready and willing to participate in the kitchen.

Continue to incorporate bilateral coordination skills into your time together in the kitchen. Perhaps your child can help you make cookies, pouring dry ingredients from the measuring cup into the mixing bowl. Roll out the cookie dough with a rolling pin and press the cookie cutters firmly into the dough. Later, clap your hands together and watch the flour clouds puff up over the counter! Be careful not to place the cookie cutter more often in one hand than the other—this is not the time to establish hand dominance. In fact, occupational therapists prefer to see hand dominance in children closer to age three. A preference for one hand over the other prior to age three indicates that your toddler's brain growth could be imbalanced, and you want to exercise both hemispheres.

Toddlers who are comfortable using both sides of their bodies (and thus both sides of their brains) are more comfortable exploring their environment, especially at mealtimes. These active "growing time" periods are essential for learning and brain development. Ensuring that "eating time" and "growing time" are scheduled throughout the day (see page 99) means that you're parenting with consistency and proactively preparing your child for each conquest in motor skills.

FINE MOTOR DEVELOPMENT

- Why some toddlers hesitate to interact with new foods and what to do about it
- Why some toddlers pick up food and toss it, and what to do about that
- Parenting Proactively: Anticipate Your Child's Next Move

Typical Development: Fine Motor Skills

At sixteen months of age, your toddler is beginning to point to pictures in books and to objects or people in her environment. Her pincer grasp is perfected. She's a pro at pouring water from one container to another. She's holding her own cup, spoon, and fork with ease by age two. For many kids, this is the stage where you might say, "Those are some very fine 'fine motor skills'!" All the more reason for your child to show off those new skills by throwing utensils over the edge of the high chair tray, pitching food at Daddy's head, and pouring her open cup of milk all over her plate of spaghetti.

Coach Mel's Tip: What to Do When Toddlers Throw Utensils or Food

When toddlers begin to throw things from the high chair, they are practicing the principle of cause and effect: Drop the spoon, Mommy picks it up. Toss chicken on the floor, the dog comes running. Throw food at Daddy, and everybody laughs! It's hard to resist responding at first, but try your best to give any undesirable behavior very little attention. It only reinforces that behavior and ensures that it will occur again and again.

Instead, give your toddler something better to do with the spoon, the cup, or the food being tossed. Try to limit utensils to just three. Three spoons means the parent gets one and the child gets two at the beginning of the meal. Whenever one gets tossed over the edge, just ignore it. Don't even look down. If all three spoons hit the floor, just eat with hands. Over time, your toddler will learn that you simply don't pick up spoons and he'll be much less likely to intentionally feed the floor. When a spoon slips accidently, it's fine to offer another one—but again, only three spoons at the table.

Throwing cups is another behavior that always gets a big reaction, even if it's just a loud crash on the floor! Calmly yet slyly intercept the cup as you sense that it's about to fly. Using hand-over-hand guidance, help your child place the cup in a marked spot on the high chair tray. Many trays have an indentation in the corner just for holding the cup, or you can place a sticker to mark the spot where the cup should land after taking a drink. Smile and say, "Your cup goes here!" and then praise her. That's the desired behavior and the one that you want to reinforce until it becomes habit.

Likewise, give your child something better to do with the broccoli than throw it. Provide a bowl that sticks to the tray or use a partitioned plate and reserve an empty spot just for moving food. When you sense that he's picking up the veggie in order to dump it for the dog, move stealthily without much reaction. Provide hand-over-hand guidance while saying, "You can put your broccoli in this bowl." Our favorite bowl that sticks is actually a bowl and placemat all in one made by ezpzfun.com and it's appropriately called the Happy Mat!

If your child loves to chuck the plate, simply keep all food on the tray for a while or use the Happy Mat to hold his food. Most importantly, engage in positive interactions with your toddler, using the food as props. "This broccoli looks like a little tree and I'm going to bite off all the leaves! *Crunch!*" or "Let's line up the carrot sticks and make a train track on your tray." Give kids something fun to do with the food! In the meantime, when utensils or food get pitched, your job is to be unimpressed.

 After letting your toddler explore, you can anticipate undesired behavior and redirect your toddler to different behavior. Remember, kids are little scientists, constantly testing cause and effect. Your job is to let them learn and, when necessary, give them a new experiment that piques their curiosity.

How to Guide Your Child: Fine Motor Skills

When children demonstrate a delay in fine motor skills, it can impact their willingness to interact with all the different textures, shapes, and aspects of the new foods that you're offering. You can boost your sixteen- to twenty-four-month-old's fine motor skills by:

- Encouraging gross motor play that strengthens the trunk, arms, and hands, such as crawling, "wheelbarrows," and climbing up and down playground equipment.

- Playing with your child by building block towers and stringing large beads, and be sure to include shape sorters and ring stackers. Watch how your child rotates his wrist to get each piece in the correct spot. Wrist rotation is necessary for using a spoon and a fork with minimal spilling.

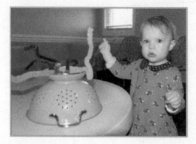 Montessori catalogs are great places to find materials to practice fine motor skills, but many of these activities can also be made from common household objects. For instance, while you're cooking, give your toddler a colander with holes (not slits). Give her a stack of pipe cleaners that are bent in different configurations and show her how to put the end of the pipe cleaner into the holes. Soon she will create a forest of pipe cleaners!

- Playing in food! Kids need to experience the various aspects of foods via all the nerves on the palms of their hands, the joints in their fingers, and their other senses, too. Think about when you're shopping for a sweater: You don't just pull it over your head and decide to buy it. No, you hold it in your hands and give it a good look. You run your hand over the knit weave, deciding if the texture is right for you. Is it soft? Is it scratchy? Is it bulky? How does the weight of it feel in your arms? Often, food exploration is dependent on how well a child can use his fine motor skills and sensory system to take the next step: tasting that brand-new food.

 If you're noticing that your child's development is lagging even a tiny bit, be sure to consult with your pediatrician, who may refer your child for an evaluation where you'll learn more tips on how to get him back on track with his peers.

Coach Mel's Tip: Four Games to Get Kids to Interact with Certain Foods

As noted in chapter 5, food exploration begins with the parent learning to tolerate their child's messy hands and face! Especially for the hesitant eater, this may be where a child needs to start. Our palms and fingers are rich with nerve endings, but the mouth has even more. Playing with food provides the child with information about a food's size, texture, temperature, and changing properties. Little hands squish and squash, pat and roll, or just pick up and let go—splat!

Here are three silly ways to play with food. Give it a try: Some of that food just may end up in your child's mouth in the process. But if it doesn't, don't worry. Learning to be an adventurous eater takes time and the most important part of the journey is keeping it fun!

1. Pudding Car Wash: For kids who can't tolerate the feel of purees, learning to play in a consistently smooth puree, like chocolate pudding, is the preliminary step to eventually playing in more textured foods, like mashed cauliflower. The key is *water*. Most kids who hate to get messy enjoy water play, for obvious reasons. If they can't tolerate water play, then that's the place to start, and eventually they will progress to pudding. You'll need:

- Chocolate pudding

- Cookie sheet

- Small toy cars

- 2 large bowls—one filled with water and soap bubbles, and the other with clean water

It's simple! Dump some "mud" (chocolate pudding) on the cookie sheet and you now have a "muddy run raceway" to drive through until the cars are coated! Pushing a toy car through the mud is much easier than playing in the mud with bare hands. The bigger the car, the easier it is for kids to tolerate the sensation, because less mud gets on the hesitant child's hand. Plop the car in the "wash" (the soap bubble water) and then fish it out. Plop it in the clear water and begin again. The water adds a bit of relief for the kids who are sensitive, but the fun of driving the cars through the mud provides the reinforcement for getting messy. Warning: This could go on all day—kids quickly learn to love it! To add variety, use plastic animals and wash the entire zoo![41]

2. Ice Pop Stir Sticks: For kids who cannot tolerate icy-cold in their mouths, here's a way to take off the chill. There is a significant difference between "straight-from-the-freezer frozen" and just icy-cold. Take a fruity ice pop on a stick and dip it in cool water. The surface of the ice pop immediately begins to melt. Now, when your kiddo takes a lick, she'll only lick off flavored cold water. Keep stirring the pop in the water and the water becomes darker and more flavorful. Let kids taste the water with a skinny straw. Coffee stirrers work as well as a tiny straw, because the narrow diameter of the stirrer allows just the tiniest taste to land on the tongue.[42]

3. Handprint Animal Pictures: Coach Mel always shudders when she observes kids in day care having to make "handprint" pictures if she knows they have sensory challenges, including tactile defensiveness. This is a term used to describe a child's reaction to touch and all the related sensations: texture, temperature, etc. As one example, many children cannot tolerate the "feel" of anything wet. The well-meaning teacher pushes the child's hand into a paper plate of paint before pressing it onto a piece of construction paper to make the infamous handprint, which is later transformed into an animal to be displayed in the classroom. Another variation that some kids find difficult to tolerate is getting the hand painted with a tickly paintbrush. That can be *very* upsetting for a child who doesn't like to get messy.

Instead, let the teacher make her own handprint, then encourage the child to use the tip of his index finger or the side of his thumb to make the eye of the handprint animal. That's the part of the hand where most kids are willing to tolerate a little mess. Think about how you pick up a slimy worm on the sidewalk: You snag it with just the tip of your index finger and the side of your thumb and then toss it quickly back into your garden. That quick release is key—kids need that, too. Over time, they'll work their way up to making an entire zoo of handprint pictures![43]

4. **Broccoli Basketball:** When enjoying a meal at the table together, consider that your child may need to first experience a food by using the very tip of his finger, then the side of his thumb, and picking it up with a quick release. Encourage this natural process by asking for a morsel of the food from his plate, so he can quickly pick it up and release it onto your plate. Or, create silly games that encourage interactions with the non-preferred food, like broccoli basketball. Hold a cup and let him drop the broccoli into the cup with a quick release. Over time, move the cup slowly through the air, being silly and fun, while your toddler holds the broccoli, waiting for the cup to float closer so he can make a basket. (Remember, we're not throwing broccoli; we are dropping it in the basket.) Now, you have a child who is holding broccoli and giggling.

 There are times for manners at the table and times to be silly. We're enthusiastic about using silly games to encourage young kids to interact with new foods. At this early age, fun is the number one priority and it leads to adventurous eating. If the silliness gets in the way of eating, save it for time away from the table using food crafts and food science activities to keep the sense of joy a bit more contained.

ORAL MOTOR SKILL DEVELOPMENT

- How to teach open-cup drinking
- Why some kids stuff their cheeks and how to change that
- Making food safe for toddlers

By sixteen months of age, your toddler has developed a mature swallow pattern. He moves his tongue all around the inside of his mouth, intentionally using it to place food on his brand new teeth and retrieve the chewed food in order to be swallowed. (See tooth eruption chart.) He's biting into large pieces of food. His chew is becoming more rotary in nature, similar to the way adults chew. In fact, his jaw, lips, and tongue begin to move independently from each other, and by age two, he's almost mastered the ability to dissociate jaw, lip, and tongue movements. This is the perfect time to focus his current level of superb motor development on one easy-to-teach task: open-cup drinking.

UPPER TEETH	ERUPT	SHED
Central Incisor	8 to 12 months	6 to 7 years
Lateral Incisor	9 to 13 months	7 to 8 years
Canine	16 to 22 months	10 to 12 years
First Molar	13 to 19 months	9 to 11 years
Second Molar	25 to 33 months	10 to 12 years

LOWER TEETH	ERUPT	SHED
Second Molar	23 to 31 months	10 to 12 years
First Molar	14 to 18 months	9 to 11 years
Canine	17 to 23 months	9 to 12 years
Lateral Incisor	10 to 16 months	7 to 8 years
Central Incisor	6 to 10 months	6 to 7 years

How to Guide Your Child: Oral Motor Skills

The key to teaching a child to drink from an open cup is to break it into simple steps and master one skill at a time. Coach Mel prefers to use glass baby food jars for this task and will sometimes wrap a few wide rubber bands around the glass so that the child has a better grip. The four-ounce jars are the ideal size for little hands, and the mouth of the jar is the perfect circumference to fit in the corners of a toddler's mouth. Too often, parents use their own adult-size glass to offer sips to a child, but think about it—that's like you and me drinking from a bucket. Fill the jar with water to where the lid of the jar screws on. Thanks to the weight of it filled almost to the brim, kids can feel the cup in their hands much better. Add a splash of color with a dark-colored juice so your child can easily see the surface of the water.

Now, you're ready to teach four simple steps to drinking from an open cup:

1. Using hand-over-hand guidance, help your child lift the cup straight up from the table and set it back down. Practice several times, repeating the mantra, "Lift up, set down, stay dry." (See figure 1.)

2. Add a new step to the end of this sequence. Bring the cup to the child's lips and have her sip, but never tilt. Your toddler will be able to do this because she can see the surface of the water and it's filled high enough that there is no need to tip. Your child may have practiced tipping before (and pouring water down the front of her shirt). The mantra and sequence is now, "Lift up, cup to lips, sip, set down, stay dry." Practice as many times as needed, replenishing the water to ensure there is no need to tilt the cup. (See figure 2.)

3. Now that step 2 is mastered, you're ready to teach the tilt-up, and more importantly, if you want to avoid a waterfall, it's time to teach the tilt-down. Kids who spent months drinking from a sippy cup have trouble with this stage, because they are used to sipping and then pulling the cup away without immediately tipping it back down. To teach the tilt-down, Coach Mel says, "Put your cup on your tummy," as she points to her entire chest and belly area. Kids at this age seem to think that "tummy" means anything between shoulders and hips. Now the mantra and sequence is as follows: "Lift up, cup to lips, sip, cup on your tummy." Repeat several times, but don't refill the glass. As the surface of the liquid lowers with each sip, the child will naturally tilt the glass slightly to sip. The key is the final step, "Put the cup on your tummy," which automatically causes the child to tilt the cup down. (See figure 3.)

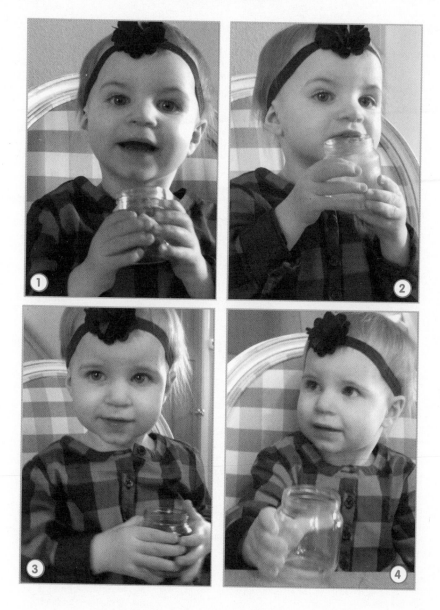

4. Once your toddler has learned to put the edge of the cup on her tummy, she can either rest it there until drinking again or follow through by placing it back on the table. (See figure 4.)

FOODS THAT CAN CAUSE CHOKING

Hard or Round Foods That Get Stuck in the Windpipe or the Lungs	Stringy or Sticky Foods That Bind Together in the Windpipe or the Lungs	Squishy Foods That Wedge in the Windpipe or the Lungs
whole grapes, olives, cherries	raisins	marshmallows
whole nuts larger than a pea	stringy meats	too much nut butter, alone or on bread
chunks of hot dogs, sausages, hard cheeses	chunks of celery; citrus segments with membrane attached	large pieces of soft rolls, breads
food with seeds, such as an orange slice	chunks of bell pepper	popcorn
hard candies	gummy candies, caramels	gummy candies, chewing gum

ADAPTATIONS TO MAKE THESE FOODS SAFER FOR TODDLERS

Hard or Round Foods	Stringy or Sticky Foods	Squishy Foods
• Cut softer round foods into pea-sized or kidney-bean-sized portions. • Avoid hard candies completely. • Remove all seeds before serving fruits. • Chop nuts to pea-size.	• Serve raisins and other small, sticky foods one piece at time. • Cut chewy candies into kidney bean-sized pieces and dole out one at a time (or ideally delay introducing them until after age three.) Each piece should be swallowed individually. • Cut stringy meats or vegetables into kidney bean-sized pieces or very narrow slivers.	• Cut squishy foods into pea- or kidney-bean-sized pieces, serving just one at a time until each individual piece is swallowed. • Popcorn is especially dangerous; be careful to only choose one piece and inspect it for a hard kernel. • Teach your child to bite larger pieces of bread and tear them off using the fringe method (see Maya's Story, page 119). • Avoid chewing gum until after age three and begin with kidney-bean-sized pieces at that time.

Dr. Yum's Tip: Watch Out for Choking
Never take your eyes off toddlers when they are eating! Remember, choking typically has no sound, so you'll only *see* choking; you won't necessarily hear it.

··

MAYA'S STORY:
No More Chipmunk Cheeks

It's common for toddlers to stuff their cheeks with food, just like a chipmunk. Problem is, once they've packed it in there, they aren't quite sure how to swallow it! This was a consistent issue for little Maya, and her mother was concerned that Maya would choke on the huge, gummy pieces of food lodged in her chipmunk cheeks.

Children often stuff because they have poor awareness in their mouths (due to inadequate proprioception). The more they stuff, the more signals travel to the brain that say, "*Now* I can feel that food in my mouth!" Sometimes they stuff until they have to pull out the chewed-up food (gross!), and sometimes they keep eating, allowing smaller pieces of food to be swallowed while the stored gummy mess prevents any decent amount from reaching their belly. This habit can be a choking hazard and can cause weight loss and cavities.

Coach Mel encouraged Maya's mom to "wake up" Maya's mouth by brushing her teeth, gums, tongue, and even the inside of her cheeks with a soft toothbrush before every meal. They did it as part of their mealtime routine, right after washing hands. That stimulation before eating alerts the brain to pay attention to what's about to happen in the mouth.

Maya's mom and Coach Mel also focused on teaching Maya to bite finger foods, like a sandwich, correctly. Whenever a child is having an issue with food, think about the steps it takes to eat that food. What step is that child missing? Think about how you eat a sandwich: You bite, tear with your teeth, and pull the sandwich away from your mouth. Maya was biting, tearing, and stuffing. Therefore, the step to teach is "pulling it away after tearing."

Each day, Maya's mother took clean kitchen shears and cut small fringe about a half-inch apart around the edge of Maya's peanut butter and jelly sandwich. (You may opt to remove the crust.) That fringe helped Maya tear off a bite easily, which led to the next step: "Pull it away!" When teaching children, always exaggerate the step you want them to focus on. For Maya, we chanted as we ate together, "Take a bite and *PULL IT AWAYYYYYYY!*" as we dramatically pulled our sandwiches away from our mouths, as if to blow a great big sandwich kiss across the table. This gave Maya a moment to chew and swallow the tiny piece, making it impossible for her to pocket it in her cheek. With repeated practice, Maya learned the step she had been missing and quit stuffing her mouth. After a while, she became more aware of what was in her mouth and no longer needed to brush her teeth before meals. (But brushing *after* is always a good idea!)

....

Cognitive Skills Related to Feeding

In these eight short months, you'll see new cognitive skills emerge in your little one, especially at mealtimes. She is now trying to feed you or perhaps her teddy bear with a spoon, because she understands that objects have specific purposes. Yet, she'll use that same spoon as a tool to retrieve a pea that has rolled just out of reach. She perseveres with problem solving more than in the past and demonstrates a wider range of emotions, including frustration when she can't quite seem to figure it out. When she is successful, she takes pride in it and beams, often looking at you to communicate with her eyes: "Hey, did you see that? I did that all by myself!"

ENGAGING YOUR TODDLER

- Simple yet fun ways kids can feel helpful
- The toddler appetite: Unpredictable twists and turns
- Mixing it up: Keeping familiar foods fun

Activities to Make the Kitchen Fun for Your Toddler

You are now at the point where your child may actually start to "help" you in the kitchen. Her fine and gross motor skills are developed enough that she can be given simple cooking and cleanup chores. The tasks you give your child now set the stage for the lasting memories your family will build as you spend time together in the kitchen. These activities will build skills and confidence and lay the foundation for future cooking skills and an interest in healthy food:

1. Washing: Give your child a shallow basin of water to wash produce, like leafy greens or grapes. Provide a scrub brush or toothbrush to scrub vegetables like potatoes or carrots. Give her a kitchen towel to put the clean produce on when she is done.

2. Tearing: A great way to introduce leafy greens is to let your toddler tear the greens into smaller pieces. Have fun with different colors of leaves, like purple kale or rainbow chard.

3. Pouring: Begin to practice pouring with dry foods, like beans. Use two small cups with spouts to pour the beans back and forth. Encourage a two-handed pour, with one hand on the handle and the other hand on the front of the cup for stability. Place a tray under the cups to catch any spills. Advance to thicker liquids like batter, and later, to thin liquids.

4. Stirring: Give kids a small whisk or spoon and a bowl to practice stirring. Keep the food level in the bowl low at first and, as they get better, show kids how to press the spoon against the bowl to prevent spills. Again, a tray or grippy mat under the bowl may create more stability and make for easier cleanup.

5. Wiping: Give your toddler a moist sponge and show him how to wipe up his cooking space.

6. Sweeping: Kid-sized brooms and mops can sweep up real food messes or piles of colorful crumpled tissue paper. This activity teaches cleanup skills and also develops gross motor strength.

Coach Mel's Tip: Bring Kids Up to the Counter

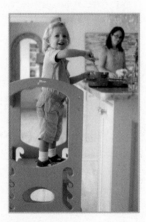

Bringing kids up to counter height may make participation easier for your toddler. The Learning Tower, by Little Partners, is a wonderful, safe platform that can be adjusted for your child's height. It can be used from toddler years to school age, making it a great investment for many years of cooking with kids.

When Familiar Food Gets Boring

For the most part, your child is now eating *almost* all of the foods that you're eating. You may start to notice his appetite becoming more unpredictable. You also may start to notice him refusing foods that he once ate happily. Don't despair—this phase will pass. Follow the parenting principles outlined in chapter 1 that focus on body, brain, and soul.

By age two, your toddler has made rapid advancements in gross motor and fine motor skills, as well as cognitive skills. You'll observe that his play is becoming more complex. His emotions and moods are just as complicated—and they may change from one moment to the next. As your child makes strides in all of these areas, the world *away* from the mealtime table is so much more interesting. If you want your child to be just as interested in staying at the table and focusing on food, it's time to change it up and keep the fun in feeding. Here are four tips to get toddlers interacting with familiar foods by making those "same old" foods more appealing and, in essence, "new."

Change up the color: Cauliflower, carrots, bell peppers, and tomatoes are just a few veggies that come in unique colors. Try introducing new colors, such as orange cauliflower interspersed in a bowl of familiar white cauliflower.

Miniaturize: Funny how kids love *tiny*! Food is much more approachable when it's made smaller. For a food that's drifting into the "been there, ate that" category, changing the size can make all the difference. Use small, child-safe food cutters like FunBites to create bite-size pieces in all sorts of shapes, like triangles and hearts.

Serve samples: Mini-muffin tins are the perfect sampling dishes, offering another way to miniaturize and not overwhelm a toddler. Remember, less is more at this stage. It's best to use the tins that have only six muffin cups. If your toddler is hesitant, you might start with filling just three with samples, or fill all six if that fits your toddler's personality.

Play with food: It's worth repeating! If you want your child to explore what's on his plate, make food appealing by making it playful. Stack cheese cubes, "paint" your plate with yogurt, or make squishy sounds with cherry tomatoes. As you have fun, you may find that the food may or may not make its way into your toddler's little mouth. But he's sitting at the table, interacting with food, and giggling with you. Parent joyfully! You may not remember the bite of carrots, but you'll always remember the joy that you brought to the dinner table. Best of all, your child will, too.

Dr. Yum's Tip: Hunger Can Be Helpful

In the first year of life, there is a period of rapid growth in both weight and body length. During the second year, growth is much more gradual. As a result, your toddler may have much less of an appetite than he did when he was a baby. It's common to see toddlers eat sporadically, sometimes eating very little for a meal or several meals, and then eating more voraciously for the next few meals.

If your toddler does not eat the foods you offer, resist the urge to fill him up with empty calories, like gummy snacks and crackers. Realize your child has his own hunger cues and already has a natural understanding of how much food his body needs. Present a variety of whole foods, some familiar and some he is still practicing, and know that for the most part toddlers will eat enough to keep going and growing.

Toddlers can sometimes eat very little, and it's a natural phase. When your child is going through periods of having less appetite, don't let your own fear get in the way of your plan. Trust what you know, and use your child's checkups (at eighteen and twenty-four months) to review her growth chart and confirm that she is growing appropriately. Continue to offer healthy whole foods, knowing that your child is eating what she needs to grow.

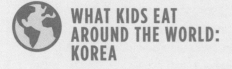

WHAT KIDS EAT AROUND THE WORLD: KOREA

Kimchi is a fermented vegetable dish typically made with Chinese cabbage, radish, cucumbers, onions, garlic, and lots of red chili powder. Korean toddlers are first offered this dish in a milder form, which may be one of the reasons they become accustomed to Korean foods' famously bold and spicy flavors so early. Kimbab, similar to Japanese sushi rolls, is another milder favorite that is made from sesame oil, rice, and vegetables wrapped in seaweed sheets, with different fillers like eggs, cucumber, kimchi, or spinach.

Making your own kimbab is fun and can be a great project for your family. Use traditional Korean ingredients or roll kimbab with some of your own favorites.

Kimbab

Here is a chance to introduce familiar foods in a new way. Let your child use favorite ingredients and let her roll the kimbab with your guiding hands. When serving this to a toddler, cut each slice into smaller bites, making it easier to manage.

A bamboo mat for rolling sushi is helpful to make this recipe, but not necessary. Try a clean kitchen towel as another option.
1 cup cooked brown or white sticky rice
1 pack (10 sheets) roasted seaweed sheets (nori)

For the filling
Adjust the amounts according to your family's tastes. You might like more carrots than eggs—it's up to you! Most importantly have fun making it together! Have a small amount of each option so that your kids still experience making the kimbab and can choose their own combination of filling.

Veggies like green onions, carrots, avocado, and/or peeled
  cucumber, cut into long, thin strips
Cooked spinach, sautéed until wilted with a drizzle of sesame oil
Favorite meats or fish, cut into strips
Fried or scrambled egg

1. Place a sheet of seaweed paper on a bamboo sushi-rolling mat, smooth side down, so that the lines on the paper are parallel to lines on the mat. If you're making smaller rolls, you can cut or tear off the top third of the sheet of nori. Larger rolls can be made with the whole sheet.

2. When the rice is cool enough to handle, using slightly wet hands or a silicone spatula, carefully spread a thin layer of rice onto the seaweed, coming as close as possible to the side edges and about 1 inch from the top and bottom edges.

3. Add the filling. Choose a combination of meat or seafood, eggs, and/or veggies and lay them horizontally across the rice. Using the mat to guide you, roll the paper, rice, meat, and veggies into a tight roll, keeping ingredients in place with your fingers. The mat helps to create an even roll, but this can be done without a mat as well. Seal the top edge with a dab of water by running your wet finger along the edge.

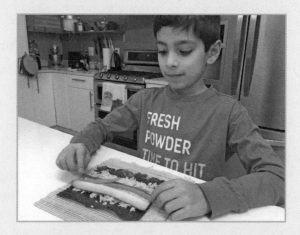

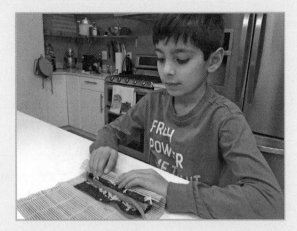

4. Let the roll rest for a few minutes and cut it into ½-inch segments. (Wiping your knife with water or sesame oil can keep it from getting sticky.) Reveal your beautiful creation! Children may enjoy dipping it in plain soy sauce or another favorite dip.

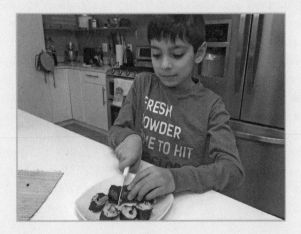

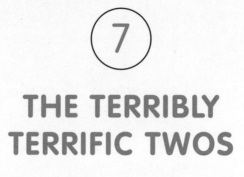

THE TERRIBLY
TERRIFIC TWOS

Ah, the two-year-old! One minute they are up and the next minute they are down, and you get to go along for the ride for the next twelve months. In the midst of the "terrible twos," most parents suspect that the trek to adventurous eating is about to get even tougher. But this is actually a great time, when a child's brain development allows for increased independence, the ability to make choices, and beginning to understand consequences. On the other hand, the two-year-old's more advanced cognitive development can present more opportunities for mealtime challenges because she's now more equipped to test her environment. In this chapter, we'll help you solve some of the more predictable challenges around mealtime routines, consistently and joyfully—even if you have to dig deep!

TYPICAL MOTOR SKILL DEVELOPMENT
IN A NUTSHELL

Your little two-year-old has mastered the gross motor, fine motor, and oral motor skills to become a super-adventurous eater. He's walking upright with improved trunk support in order for his limbs, hands, and fingers to operate with two-year-old perfection. His oral motor skills are amazing, as evidenced by his burst of two-word phrases, and his speech may reveal full sentences by age three. Speech and feeding skills often coincide with this increased mouth awareness. The power of language and continued exposure to a variety of foods leads kids to wonderful interactive experiences in and out of the kitchen. As he approaches three, your child begins to learn where food comes from and is an eager and active participant in "helping" in the kitchen.

Over the next year, you'll notice your child's oral motor skills become more refined, and by age three, your child will be eating just like a little adult. The remaining chapters will focus on behavior—and what better place to address mealtime behaviors than the terrific twos.

Cognitive Skills Related to Feeding

Over the next twelve months, you may find yourself asking, "Wow, how did she learn that?" as your two-year-old demonstrates newfound skills on a weekly basis. She is beginning to build more vocabulary and new words pop out, allowing her to make choices and let her needs be known—sometimes quite dramatically. She'll understand basic time concepts, like *"after* dinner we'll have dessert," but may not always cooperate with those statements. Until closer to age three, she won't understand good-natured teasing like "Daddy's going to eat it if you don't!" so choose your words carefully. It might get her to eat it, but it may not be a positive encounter.

In this period of rapid growth, parents often introduce the concept of color, asking, "What color is this broccoli?" and then answering their own question for their child by saying, "Green!" While that type of practice is helpful for modeling the question and answer sequence, younger two-year-olds aren't always ready to identify colors on their own. Naming the correct color is actually one of the last steps to learning color concepts ("The broccoli is green"). Matching colors and sorting them into groups is the first step. ("Broccoli, zucchini, and cucumbers are all the same color—green.")

Snack times are the perfect opportunity for this. Start with matching just two colors: Cut orange and yellow peppers into four to six strips and place them on the table with two bowls. Help your child sort the peppers, as you say "orange with orange" and "yellow with yellow," teaching her the concept of matching. Over time, you'll be able to place one orange pepper strip and one yellow pepper strip in each bowl and she'll pick up the appropriate match from the table and plop it in the correct container. Eventually, she'll be able to sort three and four different colors. Keeping the shape the same at first helps her to focus on the main theme: colors. By age three, your child will be able to sort multiple vegetables as the two of you make a beautiful salad. She'll likely hold up a piece of broccoli and declare, "It's green!" This type of cognitive skill building is not only educational, but also gets kids interacting with food. Don't be surprised when you hear a "crunch" in the midst of all this sorting.

During this period of rapid cognitive growth your two-year-old becomes more independent. She is beginning to understand that she is truly a different being than you and that she has considerable control over your actions and behaviors. This is a time where parenting with consistency is more important than ever, so that toddlers realize that while they have independence, there are still rules that they must learn.

 Doesn't it seem like the two-year-old spends much of the day being demanding? It can be easy for us as parents to be equally frustrated. However, if you step into his shoes for a moment, you can parent compassionately. Imagine being in a foreign country and only being able to speak in limited, short phrases. You have a myriad of wants and needs and a limited number of ways to express yourself. This is essentially how he feels much of the time. With your guidance, and as his language improves, the road will get easier.

Two-year-olds are beginning to label their own feelings, including distinguishing between "sad" and "mad," even when both feelings create bucket loads of tears. Have you ever noticed how some two-year-olds seem to turn on the waterworks as easily as the bathroom faucet? They aren't being manipulative.

They just have significant difficulty managing their emotions, especially when tired or hungry. In the next section, we'll discuss how easy it is to unintentionally reinforce those mood swings and condition a child to overreact to the slightest change or smallest disappointment.

MANAGING MEALTIME BEHAVIORS

- Be careful: You may be encouraging undesired behaviors in your child
- How to redirect kids who spit out or refuse food
- When spitting out food may signal a feeding disorder
- How taste testing can advance your toddler's eating habits
- Food jags and how to prevent them

Be Careful What You Reward

If you took an Intro to Psychology class, you may remember B. F. Skinner. Skinner was an American psychologist who was an expert on human behavior and coined the term "contingency of reinforcement." Coach Mel uses Skinner's principles in her work helping children learn to eat and encourages parents to use the same principles in parenting. The key to creating positive behaviors in children is to use consistent reinforcement until the behavior becomes second nature.

The younger two-year-old is aware of consequences now but may have trouble remembering exactly what that consequence was when it occurred just five minutes ago. Her attention to her environment is fleeting at times, and she's easily distracted. This impacts safety: She isn't likely to remember that you just said "No!" when she ran into your neighborhood street, and when she is distracted she'll wander into the street again. It's easy to be consistent when it comes to safety habits—in the case of running into the street, it is never, ever OK. Yet consistency around mealtime behaviors may not always be practiced. Is that a big deal? Yep—and here's why.

Contingency of reinforcement is a term used to describe the

relationship between three components: (1) The occasion or inci-dence that cues the behavior; (2) The behavior itself; (3) The con-sequences following the behavior.[44] Keep in mind that a behavior can be desired (your child happily eats carrots) or undesired (your child spits carrots in your face). No matter which one, the ulti-mate question is: What happened just before and just after the behavior? The behavior of spitting is a good example: What hap-pened just before he spit those carrots and then what happened after he spit them in your face? Did you make a scene or break out laughing? Or did you calmly wipe the carrots off your face and simply turn away? That minimal reaction is actually a "con-sequence," and when it comes to behaviors like spitting, it's a good one. Here's why.

Throughout our days of parenting, you and your child are exchanging millions of behaviors and reactions (consequences) to those behaviors. As mentioned above, parents tend to be most consistent reinforcing the desired behaviors when it comes to safety. For example, when you put your screaming toddler in his car seat and buckle him up, you give the protests very minimal attention, if any at all. There is not an option when riding in a car other than being in the car seat. Your toddler quickly learns that and soon learns to quit fussing about getting buckled in. The occasion that cued the fussing was likely you picking him up and putting him in the car seat. The behavior was the crying. The consequence was "ignoring" and buckling him in anyway. By ignoring the crying, you helped that behavior fade away, and now he can travel in his seat like a champ! That's parenting using Skinner's model. Most importantly, what makes it work so well is *parenting with consistency.*

Let's talk about when it doesn't work in your favor, when there is no consistency. By consistent, we mean that the same reaction needs to occur at least 80 percent of the time. If you're establish-ing a new rule, then we suggest 100 percent consistency during the learning process and 80 percent consistency after the rule has been established and practiced. Consistency creates habits—good and bad habits. Sometimes in life, it's hard to be consistent.

Picture this: You're in the checkout lane at the grocery store and your two-year-old is starting to melt down. She spies the candy intentionally displayed at the checkout line for that impulsive, last-minute purchase. She begins to whine, "Candy pwease," and you respond, "No sweetie, we're almost done here and then we are going home for some yummy lunch." But she's cranky and tired and her behavior escalates: *"Want CANDY*!!!!" She starts to cry.

Now, everyone is staring at you, from the clerk behind the counter to the impatient businessman standing in line behind you. "Me *WANT CANDY!*" she declares loudly, sobbing. "Fine! Here! Just stop crying!" you whisper under your breath, grabbing the nearest M&Ms and pushing it into her little hands. Magically, the crying stops. Feeling relieved and guilty all at the same time, you know what you were supposed to do. Let her cry and stay consistent with "no." But oh, the pressure—and those people staring at you with their "judgy eyes." Hey, we get it. We really do. Here's the problem: Do that a few more times and you've now got a toddler who doesn't just whine when she sees candy, she immediately jumps to screaming, *"ME WANT CANDY!"* and having a full-fledged meltdown. That's because that was the behavior that was reinforced. That's what got her candy.

When you have a two-year-old, parenting with consistency is vital in order to manage mealtime behaviors. Be careful what behaviors you reinforce through unintentional consequences, like giving in when your child's behavior escalates. When you give in even a few times, your child will quickly learn to rev up her behavior in order to get what she wants. Without realizing it, you can consistently reinforce *undesired* behaviors—like whining—or you can be intentionally consistent by not responding and the whining will fade away. Giving your child the words she can use for next time is helpful. Readdress this when your child has calmed down and model the words by parenting with compassion.

Spitting Out Food

Keep that same scenario in mind, whether you're trying to teach a desired behavior or stop an undesired behavior from occurring again. Be careful how you react and pay attention to what you may have accidently reinforced. The first time a child intentionally and forcefully spits out food, it may be impossible not to react in some manner. But keep your response as boring as possible. The interesting thing about consequences is that *doing nothing* is still a consequence. Your job is to be unimpressed. (Spitting out food in a controlled manner or pulling out food for safety reasons when the piece is just too big is different. A casual, "Yep, that piece is too big. Good idea to take it out and bite it again," is sufficient to reinforce that behavior.)

When kids chew and then spit out food because they don't want to swallow it, it can be a hard habit to break. For children with oral motor delays or other reasons to be in feeding therapy, they may not be able to propel the food back to be swallowed.

 Coach Mel's Tip: Avoid Using a Spit Cup
It's important to note that some children in feeding therapy are encouraged to use a cup to spit into, rather than spitting food onto their plate. Coach Mel prefers not to use that strategy in her feeding therapy practice and it's also not something she typically recommends for children. When a cup is present just for this purpose, it's a visual reminder to "spit here" and cues the child to think about spitting. Because this book is not a detailed "how-to" of feeding therapy techniques, we won't cover all the pros and cons here. What we will provide are alternatives and strategies for the typical child to learn to swallow food rather than spit.

You may notice your child spitting out food when it is too hot, too chewy, too big, or a mixed texture that he's having trouble managing. Kids may spit out certain foods when they have a runny nose. The mucous makes it uncomfortable to swallow certain foods. Teething and earaches also contribute to spitting because it's painful to swallow some foods.

Kids who have developmental delays spit out food for a variety of reasons and should be assessed by a qualified speech-language pathologist who specializes in swallowing and feeding disorders. Other team members may be an integral part of the evaluation process.

CLOSER LOOK:
Swallowing Disorders in Children

Dysphagia (pronounced dis-FAY-juh or dis-FAH-juh), or difficulty swallowing, is a medical condition and often occurs in conjunction with a feeding disorder. According to the American Speech-Language-Hearing Association (ASHA), the swallowing process can be divided into three distinct stages:[45]

1. Oral phase: sucking, chewing, and moving food or liquid into the throat

2. Pharyngeal phase: starting the swallow, squeezing food down the throat, and closing off the airway to prevent food or liquid from entering the airway (aspiration) or to prevent choking

3. Esophageal phase: relaxing and tightening the openings at the top and bottom of the feeding tube in the throat (esophagus) and squeezing food through the esophagus into the stomach.

Some certified speech-language pathologists (SLPs) receive specialized training in the assessment and treatment of swallowing disorders. Remember, picky eating may be more than just a phase. Follow your instincts and talk to your pediatrician, who may refer you for specialized assessment by a qualified SLP.

How to Stop the Spitting

The best way to stop the spitting is to give it very little attention when it begins to occur. This should limit spitting to only times when it's necessary and not encourage repetitive spitting for entertainment or attention. But if spitting has become the new dinnertime drama, try these techniques:

1. Watch to ensure that your child is not taking too big of a bite and/or stuffing his cheeks. Keep bites manageable (the size of a dime) even if you have to cut up pieces for him.
2. Encourage your child to put the piece of food on his molars rather than placing the piece at the very front of the mouth. This encourages immediate chewing and the food is closer to the back of the throat for immediate swallowing. Food chewed with the front teeth is more likely to be spit out.
3. As your child begins to chew, teach him to reach for his cup and straw. Taking a sip of water via a straw washes down the chewed food quite easily.
4. Be sure that your child is hungry for meals. When kids want to taste food but aren't hungry enough to go to the trouble of swallowing, they will often spit after chewing.

When Kids Refuse to Eat

By now, you have a good idea of what your child is capable of eating and what she likes and dislikes. Try to offer small samplings of preferred and nonpreferred foods, along with foods that are just "so-so" for your child's palate. Offering options, whether via family-style serving or via a pre-plated meal continues to expose your child to all types of foods, and when there is no pressure to eat it, you'll find that over time, she becomes more curious about tasting it.

Family-style servings, where the entrée and side dishes are presented on platters or large bowls and passed around the

table, allow people to help themselves to each dish. It provides the opportunity for even the most hesitant eater to
experience the sight and smell of the food. This method is
ideal for some families and adds to the social atmosphere of
sharing at meals. Repeated exposure to the same foods,
especially if the child is responsible for serving everyone's
plates, may be helpful if a child is at the stage where they
need to experience food at the most basic level. Other family
members can cue the child, "Oh, more green beans for me,
please," while he dishes up the plates, thus providing the
opportunity to interact with the new foods over and over.
From the day you introduce family-style serving, make a
rule that everyone gets a little bit of each food on his plate.
It's up to the individual if she wants to eat it.[46]

Pre-plated servings: Another option is to simply dish up the
child's plate and serve it to him. It's not always possible or
convenient to do family-style servings. If your child fusses
or negatively reacts to anything on his plate, simply state the
fact and move on. "Yep, we've got asparagus on our plate
today." The sooner your child registers that this is no big
deal, communicated by your nonchalant attitude, the
quicker the negative response will fade away. The first step
is just tolerating it on the plate; tasting comes later.

Taste Testing

Tasting new foods can be a regular part of your child's life by
making it special. Make it a part of your day that kids look forward to by calling it "Tasting Time."

"We always taste everything on our plate" may sound like the
old adage "Try one bite of everything," but tasting is very different
from biting. Whether you introduce this concept as an after-school
activity or you simply establish this rule from an early age, you're
striving to make sure it becomes a habit. Raising a confident,
adventurous eater doesn't mean he'll eat everything; it means he'll
be willing to *taste* almost anything. Consider the raw oyster. Have

your ever met anyone who saw a platter of freshly shucked raw oysters for the very first time who exclaimed, "Mmmm! I'd love to try one of those"? But children who grow up near the Chesapeake Bay are exposed to raw oysters on a frequent basis. Eventually, most kids want to try them. It's up to them if they like oysters after that, but they are willing to taste—and that's being adventurous. Expose your kids to a variety of foods early and often. Then, the rule "We taste everything on our plate" is commonplace and becomes easy to follow.

Why try to establish rules so early? Think about Yoda from *Star Wars* and his famous line to his young student, Luke. "You must unlearn what you have learned."[47] That's exactly what you'll have to do with your child. When children insist on their own separate meal at dinner rather than eat what is presented, when they fall into the habit of asking for a kids' meal when you pass by the drive-through (and you regularly give in), or when they are allowed to graze on fish-shaped crackers, they get in the habit of eating these less-than-nutritious foods. It can lead to food jags, and kids will then narrow down their repertoire to only their preferred foods. That's much harder to unlearn.

Coach Mel's Tip:
Never say "You Don't Have to Eat It"

It's common practice among feeding professionals to suggest to parents that they tell their kids, "You don't have to eat it," when the child balks at a new food on the plate. Coach Mel never does this and prefers that the parents she works with don't say it either. Why? It feels a bit dishonest. It breaks down trust, because the child knows that Coach Mel and his parents want him to try new foods. For kids not in feeding therapy, the phrase may be fine, but don't you really want your child to try new foods and then decide if he wants more? Try just stating what is happening, "Yes, we all have Brussels sprouts on our plates tonight," and change the subject. The first step is helping a child cope with the Brussels sprouts on his plate and not feeding into his anxiety about *when* he'll try it. He'll learn to taste it when he's ready.

Another alternative to stating "You don't have to eat it" is to establish taste testing from age two. If taste testing has not been established from an early age, you can U-turn and take a slightly different path and make it a regular rule at mealtimes. We have often used taste testing away from meals to build confidence and trust while keeping the experience positive and interactive. Over time, we find that we can gradually start incorporating taste testing into mealtimes until it's an established rule.

 ## Dr. Yum's Tip: Tasting Time

When Nimali started her website, DoctorYum.org, she wanted to show parents that kids could love healthy whole food. She decided it would be fun to post recipes that had ratings from real-life kids. Schoolchildren would come to her house and try new recipes, and sometimes she would even videotape them trying different foods. The idea of "Tasting Time" was born! Dr. Yum has seen how Tasting Time has worked in other places, like her cooking classes, in schools, and with patients. Here, she describes why Tasting Time has worked for her, and how it can work for your family:

Tasting Time is, ideally, separate from mealtime. Typically, the after-school period is the time I have classes and food tastings for my website. I find that having Tasting Time after school when you would serve a snack (and when kids are naturally very hungry) is ideal for trying new foods or favorite foods in new ways. When kids are asked to taste food outside of a meal, they are more likely to take the plunge. Would you want to commit to eating a whole plate of mystery food? Probably not, but you might take one taste!

I ask kids to taste with a smile on my face, with the same enthusiasm I'd ask them to smell a scratch-and-sniff sticker or listen to a cool song. I tell them, "Try this neat food and tell me how it feels in your mouth!" Present it like a fun new adventure. Research shows that children are more likely to want to try a food they dislike when it's presented with a smiling adult face.[48] So put aside your own distaste for beets and smile when you offer them to your kids.

I ask kids for feedback about food. "What does this food remind you of? Does it feel crunchy in your mouth?" Our "Yum Score" is a score system using a series of faces to help kids describe how they like a food. Keep in mind, for hesitant tasters, the Yum Score can be used for the other senses like smell. Even two-year-olds who may have limited language skills can use this tool, which we use for older kids, too. Remind kids that their taste buds need to practice. Foods that taste like "Super Yuck" can someday turn into a "Super Yum." Help kids understand that practice is important in all areas, whether it's riding a bike, playing sports, and even tasting food. In our next chapter, Coach Mel will give you some more ideas on practicing foods via tasting.

YUM SCORE

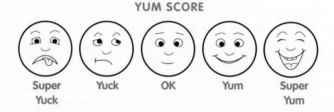

| Super Yuck | Yuck | OK | Yum | Super Yum |

We celebrate successes. If a child is not able to taste broccoli today, give him a pat on the back just for washing it, chopping it, or stirring it into the broccoli salad. Hesitant eaters get a high five for smelling a new food and encouragement so they will be closer to tasting it next time. One way to celebrate tasting is to take pictures of their tasting successes and share them with friends. This can be an inspiration to us all!

Finally, kids can encourage kids. My cooking students and taste testers often taste new foods in the company of other children. In Doctor Yum's Preschool Adventure, a preschool nutrition curriculum written by Coach Mel and me, preschoolers prepare and taste food in the classroom with other preschoolers. There is a certain amount of positive peer pressure and infectious curiosity that occurs when kids try food together. Taste food with siblings or invite friends over. One of my young patients recently told me she was going to start a "Tasting Club" with her neighborhood friends. How great is that?[49]

• •

Food Jags

Coach Mel treats kids with special needs such as autism or Down syndrome but also works with extreme picky eaters that have spiraled down to eating a few types of foods. Coach Mel even treated a child who *only* ate crunchy vegetables, like broccoli and carrots. Given his love for vegetables, it took his parents a long time to decide that such a limited diet might be a problem. No matter what the food, kids can easily get stuck in food jag: eating a very limited number of foods and strongly refusing all others. It creates havoc not only from a nutritional standpoint, but from a social aspect, too. Once their parents realize the kids are stuck, the parents feel trapped as well. It's incredibly stressful for the entire family, especially when mealtimes occur three times per day and there are only a few options for what their child will eat.[50]

Here are our "Top Ten" suggestions for preventing food jags:[51]

1. Start early. Expose baby to as many flavors and safe foods as possible.

2. Rotate, rotate, rotate. Foods, that is. Jot down what your toddler was offered and rotate foods frequently, so that new flavors reappear, regardless if your child liked (or didn't like) them on the first few encounters. This is true for kids of all ages. It's about building familiarity.

3. Food left on the plate is *not* wasted. Even if it ends up in the compost, the purpose of the food's presence on a child's plate is for her to see it, smell it, touch it, hear it, crunch it under her fork, and perhaps, taste it. So if the best she can do is pick it up and chat with you about the properties of green beans, then hurray! That's never a waste, because she's learning about a new food.

4. Offer small portions. Present small samples. *Underwhelming*—that's exactly the feeling we hope to invoke. Besides, if a sample sparks some interest and your child asks for more peas, well, that's just music to your ears, right? For hesitant eaters, it's helpful to present the foods in little ramekins, small ice cube trays, or even on the tiny tasting spoons used for samples at the ice cream shop.

5. Highlight three or four ingredients over two weeks. You can expose kids to the same three or four ingredients over the course of two weeks, while making many different recipes. Remember, get the kids involved in the recipe, so they experience the food with all of their senses. Even two-year-olds can tear fragrant basil, sprinkling it on cheese pizza. If they just want to include it as a garnish on the plate beside the pizza, that's a good start, too.

6. Focus on building relationships with food. That often doesn't begin with chewing and swallowing. Two-year-olds and preschoolers love to help in the garden, grocery shop, visit the farmers' market, and even play in food! Sounds corny (pardon the pun), but making friends with food means *getting to know* food. We often tell the kids we work with, "We are introducing your brain to Brussels sprouts. Brain, say hello to B-sprouts!"

7. Don't wait for a picky eating phase to pass. Use these strategies now. Keep them up, even through a phase of resistant eating.

8. Don't food jag on family favorites. In our fast-paced life, it's easy to grab the same thing for dinner most evenings. Because of certain preferences, are the same few foods served too often? "Let's just have pizza again—at least I know everyone will eat that." Spend time getting some new selections into the mix, knowing that after a period of adjustment your family will get used to these items.

9. Make family dinnertime less about dinner and more about family. The more a family focuses on being together, sharing tidbits of their day, and enjoying each other's company, the sweeter the atmosphere at the table. That's what family mealtimes are meant to be: a time to share our day—and that includes the youngest members of your family.

10. And the number one strategy for preventing food jags? Seek help early. If mealtimes become stressful or the aforementioned strategies seem especially challenging, that's the time to ask a feeding therapist for help. For more information, please refer to chapter 13.

Dr. Yum's Tip: How Food Jags Can Lead to Constipation and Vice Versa

Most toddlers become receptive to potty training at around twenty-seven to thirty-two months. For many toddlers with a restricted, more processed diet, fiber intake can be low, leading to constipation and painful bowel movements. While potty training, you want to set kids up for success, so pay attention to your child's bowel habits. Children should be having at least one soft bowel movement a day that is easy to pass. If bowel movements are hard, infrequent, or painful, the process of potty training can be more difficult. While working on establishing diet higher in fiber, talk to your pediatrician about ways that you can help regulate your child's bowel movements, including gentle laxatives so potty training is easier. Introducing high-fiber options like fruit and vegetable smoothies can help, too. You may notice that once your child has regular bowel movements, his appetite may increase, which can stop the cycle of food jagging.

SOCIAL ASPECTS OF FEEDING A TWO-YEAR-OLD

- Rethinking the clean plate club
- How to take dessert off its pedestal
- How to keep sugar in check
- What about kids' meals and kids' menus?

Rethinking the "Clean Plate Club"

As parents, we love our kids, and likewise we feel a strong innate need to *feed* them. This desire to feed our two-year-old can sometimes run against her natural ups and downs, especially when she does not want to eat. Remember that after age one, kids' growth plateaus and their appetite can be much smaller than what we expect.

"Joining the clean plate club" is an older parenting method that requires children to eat everything that the parents serve on their plate. No negotiating, just clean your plate. This method of parenting likely developed during a time in American history when food was scarce and it was important not to be wasteful. It's easy to see how this concept may have been passed down to our generation. Lots of folks have been brought up in this way, so what is the harm, right?

The dilemma with the clean plate club is that it doesn't allow the child to participate in deciding how much food makes him full. We instead train the child to use the visual of the empty plate to guide him to decide when to stop eating. This is a problematic scenario. The average restaurant meal has grown to epic proportions over the decades, with super-sized meals and all-you-can-eat buffets luring us into thinking that eating out is a great "value." According to the Centers for Disease Control and Prevention, since the 1950s, the size of the average hamburger and fries has tripled and the size of the average soft drink has increased 500 percent. It's not surprising that the average person weighs twenty-six more pounds than in the 1950s. Back at home, the size of plates, cups, and bowls have gotten bigger, too. In the early 1960s, the standard size of a dinner plate was ten inches, but today it has increased to twelve inches.[52] It has also been shown that the larger the bowl, the more food adults serve themselves.[53] It's not hard to imagine how these larger bowls and plates also trick us into serving more food to our kids, too.

Early in life, babies and toddlers are able to regulate intake of food using their own cues of hunger and satiety. At some point though, social cues start to influence eating behaviors and kids can be more influenced by external cues like portion size. One study of preschool-age children demonstrated that increased portion size resulted in increased food intake among five-year-olds but did not influence the amount consumed by three-year-olds.[54] Most two-year-olds still are holding on to that wonderful innate skill of knowing when to stop eating.

When we teach kids that they have to finish everything on their plate we are telling them that food needs to be eaten whether they are full or not. In our current food environment with oversized portions everywhere this parenting style is a recipe for overeating and may be one of the important factors in why childhood obesity has reached record levels.

So what to do when your two-year-old shows no interest in what you put on her plate? You can draw upon all the parenting stamps in your passport:

 Put a variety of fun foods on the table and if your toddler doesn't want to eat, take a moment to enjoy the food in other ways. *Snap* the sugar snap peas between your fingers and perhaps between your teeth. Which one is louder? Who can make the loudest snap? Start with what your child *can* do on a given day and build from there.

 If you show frustration about your child not eating enough, it can only make mealtime more difficult. Instead, know that there are times when your child will not want to eat as much as you would like, and stay focused on the bigger picture. This is a time to respect your child's instincts. He is trying to listen to his body's cues, just as you have taught him.

Most toddlers are really good at gauging how much they need to eat. The toddler appetite ebbs and flows just like yours. Be brave and trust that your parenting strategies are working.

 Remember, repetition is at the heart of food educa-tion, and you may need fifteen "Yucks" before you get to a "Yum." Throwing away some food is part of the teaching experience.

 Have a plan for when your child doesn't want to eat much. You'll still stick to your feeding schedule, but you'll plan ahead and serve a mini-meal as the next snack. Plan for that snack to be balanced and nutritious instead of grabbing a "snack food" that simply fills the belly.

 Stick to a schedule (see the feeding schedule in chap-ter 5, page 99). Adhering to a schedule will help her learn that if she doesn't eat enough, she will be hun-gry before the next opportunity to eat.

 Encourage kids as young as age two to serve them-selves by presenting meals "family-style." Family-style eating allows toddlers to practice serving food and judging how much is enough. They also learn the etiquette of ask-ing for food and passing it to others.

Why Dessert Is Not a Big Deal

Some parents may restrict treats like dessert and ban all forms of sugar, in hopes of establishing good eating habits. At first glance, this may seem like a good strategy, but there are many unwanted consequences of making too much of a big deal about dessert. By saying "no" to all desserts, you may actually be making them more appealing. Kids may end up placing more importance on dessert and lose interest in delicious whole foods that are better for them.

Sweet treats will eventually make their way to your child's mouth, whether you want them to or not. Rather than shy away from sugar, use sweet treats as a way to show your child how to build a healthy and well-rounded diet, *despite* their external environment. Dessert can have a place in your kitchen, even every day if you choose, as long as you teach kids how to manage sweets in a healthy way.

First, take sweets off their pedestal by *never* rewarding with food. When you give children sweets as a reward regularly, you're priming their neural circuitry to crave food in an unhealthy way and to eat when they are not hungry. The message also becomes that dessert is more special than other foods, making kids want it all the more.

Next, teach proportion by making dessert a regular part of your day or meal. Putting a small piece of brownie on the dinner plate shows them that dessert not a big deal, and that compared to all the other great whole foods on the plate, its proportion should be small. For older kids, dessert can be served after dinnertime, but teach proportion by limiting the serving size or rotating other sweet whole foods like fruit into the routine. Rather than serving dessert in a cereal bowl, serve it in a much smaller dessert cup, to emphasize proportion.

Also, find ways to improve the quality of the sweets you offer. Toddlers are naturally more restricted in their food choices. If you're going to allow your toddler to enjoy a treat, use the opportunity to make it from scratch with nourishing whole food ingredients that offer extra vitamins, minerals, and fiber. After all, your toddler now has the skills to help you make homemade cookies, granola bites, raw fruit desserts, and more!

There are some instances when families need to disconnect from dessert for various reasons, including trying to achieve a healthier weight or already having unhealthy habits around sweets. Families may instead choose to offer dessert during select times only, for instance, on weekends. The trick is to establish the rules about dessert and parent consistently. When kids ask for dessert on a Thursday, the answer is, "Remember the rule, we only eat dessert on weekends. I'm looking forward to those cupcakes, too!"

Dr. Yum's Tip: Be Mindful of Sugar!

As your child becomes more vocal about what he wants, he may start to demand more processed food options. These options may be well suited to the less adventurous two-year-old palate, as they are easy, bland, sweet, or salty. If you let her take the lead on what foods are offered, then you may find yourself increasingly going down the path of fruit snacks, fish-shaped crackers, and other typical toddler foods. The problem is that as we start to offer more of these processed foods, toddlers' sugar intake can skyrocket. The Environmental Working Group found in a comprehensive study of eighty thousand grocery foods that 60 percent of them had added sugar.[55] These included a wide range of foods like bologna, stuffing mix, and spaghetti sauce. The American Heart Association recommends that toddlers get no more than four added teaspoons of sugar per day (approximately twenty grams). The average toddler in America gets more than three times that! If you're sticking to healthy whole foods for the majority of your toddler's diet, then adding dessert is not a big deal. However, adding dessert to an already sugar-packed processed diet may be putting your child at risk for being overweight, having tooth decay, and a host of other diet-related symptoms.

Here is a typical toddler diet that we often observe in our interactions with children. Note that the amount of added sugar is not typically included on labels and in many instances had to be extrapolated using comparable unsweetened products.

MEAL	FOOD	TEASPOONS OF ADDED SUGAR (APPROXIMATE)
Breakfast	1 frozen blueberry breakfast waffle with 2 tablespoons breakfast syrup	5
Morning Snack	10 fish-shaped crackers and 1 pouch fruit punch	4
Lunch	1 strawberry yogurt tube, ½ peanut butter and jelly sandwich, carrot sticks with ranch dressing	5
Afternoon Snack	1 package fruit snacks and 1 packaged cereal bar	6
Dinner	4 fish sticks with ketchup 4 oz. cinnamon applesauce 6 oz. chocolate milk	7
Dessert	Store-bought ice pop	2
	TOTAL	29

THE KID'S MENU:
AVOIDING THE PATH OF LEAST RESISTANCE

We wrote this book in hopes that one day you'll never again have to utter these words: "As long we've got chicken nuggets, then my kid will eat." Avoiding the picky eater trap begins at birth, but the two-year-old brings exceptional challenges on the road to adventurous eating and it's easy to stray off course. Why? It's because your two-year-old is:

- easily influenced,
- prey to the fast-food marketing machine,
- emotionally unstable.

The next time you encounter this trifecta is when your two-year-old becomes a teenager.

One of the hidden forces that causes a parent to stray is the infamous kids' menu. It's the path of least resistance. You just want to have a nice, peaceful dinner with your spouse or your friend or gosh, just you and your child! If you're at a "sit-down" restaurant, the hostess automatically grabs a kids' menu if you're toting along anyone under twelve years old. The kids' menu is *cheap*. Your child can color on it and then take it home. When the all-too-familiar chicken nuggets or hamburger appears, it may include a toy! Sometimes there is a plastic cup that's got his favorite cartoon characters on it and there might even be free soda refills! That's called marketing—and now, they've got your kid hooked. For the marketers, it's never too early. A two-year-old is perfect: They are vulnerable and emotional. They are a marketer's dream.

Let's be real about this: We have certainly fed our own kids their fair share of chicken nuggets, mac and cheese, and French fries, just to name a few of the comfort foods that predictably appear on kids' menus day after day. We are not totally condemning the American kids' meal that is so common in fast-food chains and family restaurants. But clearly, we are not keen on eating that type of food regularly when there are other choices. Most parents know that the traditional fast-food fare is not healthy, yet "40 percent of children ages 2–11 ask their parents to go to McDonald's at least once a week, and 15 percent of preschoolers ask to go every day," as reported by the Yale Rudd Center (now located at the University of Connecticut)."[56] "Eighty-four percent of parents report taking their child ages 2–11 to a fast-food restaurant at least once in the past week."[57]

The millions of dollars spent on advertising and toys to get kids hooked on these meals certainly makes us frustrated—especially when much less is spent on marketing a culture of wellness. By hooked, we don't mean addicted. (Although there is research that suggests that food addiction may be a serious component for a subset of the pediatric population.[58] Plus, the added sugars in processed foods have been found to be addictive in lab experiments.[59]) But let's just say most kids love them.[60] The misnomer is in the name, as explained in an article in *The American Journal of Medicine* aptly titled, "The Autopsy of Chicken Nuggets Reads 'Chicken Little.'" The study concluded, "Striated muscle (chicken meat) was not the predominant component in either nugget. Fat was present in equal or greater quantities along with epithelium, bone, nerve, and connective tissue."[61] Yum! Would you like BBQ, honey mustard, or our special sauce with that?

Navigating your way around fast-food marketing would be so much easier if your two-year-old could just read a medical journal, right? But even the texture of chicken nuggets mimics that of anything else that we think of as "kids' food." Consider the other reasons that the standard kids' fare in restaurant chains seemingly makes life so much easier:[62]

1. Chewing is optional. In terms of oral motor skills, bites of chicken nuggets are a first food that even an almost toothless toddler can consume with relative ease. Simply gum, squish, and swallow. Macaroni and cheese? Oily French fries? Ditto. There's not a lot of chomping going on!

2. Kids' meals are quick. Quick to buy, quick to eat, quick to raise blood sugar, and quick to feel satisfied. We get it—part of today's hectic lifestyle is shuttling kids to and from activities, and often, mealtimes happen while riding in the minivan. Fast-food chains understand this, too, and market accordingly.

3. You know your child will eat them. But now that you're armed with new strategies and know how to introduce wholesome foods, you don't have to rely on fast food. At home, you expose your children to the same healthy food that you're eating—why should eating out be any different?

How to Ditch Kids' Menus and Kids' Meals

- Ask for the kids' menu and crayons to keep your child occupied, but skip the kid food. Begin with helping your child order from the "adult" menu, knowing that you can request adaptations to certain dishes if needed. If the prices feel too steep, order a favorite side for the kids and give them samplings of everything on your plate. The average American restaurant meal is oversized, and chances are there will be extra food on your plate that you can offer your two-year-old. Now you and your child have a new routine where tasting your food becomes a part of that routine.[63]

- If you order a salad in the drive-through, create a kid's sampling of grilled chicken cubes, sunflower seeds, mandarin oranges, or other options directly from your salad when you arrive at your destination. Request an extra packet of dressing if he likes to dip.[64]

- In today's quick-fix society, our children are losing the valuable skill of waiting. Feeling hungry and then making a snack or meal together to satisfy growling bellies is one way to practice the art of waiting. Have some precut veggies ready in the refrigerator to nibble on if waiting for the meal is too challenging. Besides, it's the perfect time to place the veggies on the counter while you're prepping the entrée because you've got hunger on your side![65]

- Dine at restaurants that serve meals family-style. For instance, in many Asian restaurants, menus are designed so that families can order larger entrées to share. This reinforces the idea that everyone eats the same food, even at a restaurant.

Coach Mel's Tip: Serve Blanched Veggies

Blanched veggies, patted dry and then chilled, hold more moisture and taste slightly sweeter to some kids. The higher moisture content makes them easier to crunch, chew, and swallow. Most blanched fresh vegetables last for several days in the refrigerator. Remember, keep presenting fresh foods so that the more common option is a healthy one, rather than the well-marketed processed foods found on many kids' menus today.[66]

AIDEN'S STORY:
Getting to a Healthier Weight

Dr. Yum visited Aiden to help with his weight. At two years old, Aiden was quite a large child and was often mistaken for a four-year-old. His mother told me that other parents were often confused by his size and seemed puzzled by his language skills and behavior, which of course reflected his actual age.

When Aiden first started to see me I was concerned about his weight, which was well over the 95th percentile (far into the obese range). I could see that his mom was having a hard time controlling him, in part because he was so big. She had zip-top bags full of snack foods like crackers, candy, and juice boxes spilling out of her diaper bag. She seemed to use food to get him to do what she wanted. "Sit up here and I'll give you a juice box. If you stay still, I'll give you a fruit snack." She also let him eat all the time and had not developed clear boundaries for when food was not offered. As his size grew more out of proportion to his age he became more difficult to control, prompting Mom to use food even more. They were stuck in an unhealthy cycle where his weight and behaviors were becoming harder to handle.

Adding to her struggle was the fact that Aiden was picky. When offered the healthy food that his parents ate, he often refused, so Mom resorted to baby food pouches, worrying that without them he would not get the nutrition he needed. After taking stock of Aiden's typical diet of juice boxes, hyperpalatable snacks, and baby food pouches, I could see that I had to give Mom some parenting tools to help her find her way and help Aiden to achieve a healthier weight.

First, we worked on getting much of the sugar out of his diet by cutting out the juice boxes. I also tried to convince her to replace the pouches with whole foods and work on a feeding schedule. After a few short months, Aiden's body mass index had plummeted. When I asked what she did, Mom reported that many of the feeding changes that we talked about were difficult, but what she was able to accomplish was not giving any more juice to her son. I showed her his growth curve and she was delighted. He was still quite high on the curve, and his diet hadn't ventured much outside of baby food, but things were surely getting better. I could tell her confidence was improving, so we explored the concept of parenting bravely and joyfully. I showed her ways that she could get Aiden onto a schedule, which helped him to be a little hungry at mealtimes and more willing to try foods. At his three-year well-child checkup, his body mass index and weight were at the 90th percentile, which was much improved over where he had started less than twelve months before. More importantly, they both were enjoying more whole foods, and his mom seemed much happier and less stressed about his health.

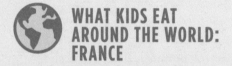 **WHAT KIDS EAT AROUND THE WORLD: FRANCE**

The French are known for their love of food, and they also take food education seriously when it comes to their children. Author Karen Le Billon experienced this firsthand when she moved her family, including two small children, from Canada to France for a year. In her book *French Kids Eat Everything*, she describes the eye-opening food experiences she and her kids had in France. She writes:

> French parents believe that their children will grow up to eat like they do: to enjoy tasting new foods, to choose a balanced diet, to eat their vegetables uncomplainingly, and to enjoy food—all food—in moderation. French parents and teachers encourage children every step of the way, believing that their children will turn out to be healthy eaters. The French government and schools support parents and teachers with an appropriate curriculum and regulations, in addition to the lessons kids learn from eating healthy school lunches. But the French also know that a true food

education starts in the home. And it begins with the belief in your children's innate capacity to eat well and your capacity to teach them to do so.[67]

Crêpes

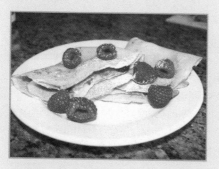

Here is a recipe for crêpes, a favorite in Dr. Yum's kitchen. She adapted this recipe from one she was given by a French exchange student years ago. Kids love being able to fill crêpes with their favorite sweet or savory fillings.

Makes about 8 crepes

2 eggs (or 4 egg whites)
1 cup milk of choice
½ cup all-purpose flour
½ cup white whole wheat flour
1 tablespoon butter, melted
1 tablespoon sugar
¼ teaspoon salt
1 tablespoon confectioners' sugar for dusting (optional)

Suggested fillings (measurements fill one crepe)

SWEET
¼ cup fresh or frozen berries
¼ cup apple, diced and sprinkled with cinnamon
1 tablespoon low-sugar jam or smashed fruit
1 tablespoon hazelnut spread

SAVORY
1 tablespoon peanut butter
1 tablespoon cream cheese

½ cup raw chopped greens sautéed with ¼ cup chopped favorite veggies and 1 teaspoon of cream cheese (creates 2 tablespoons filling)

1. Whisk together eggs and milk until combined. Add the flour, melted butter, sugar, and salt and whisk until it is the consistency of heavy cream (if too thick, add a little extra milk).

2. Coat a skillet lightly with cooking spray and heat it over medium heat. Ladle about ¼ cup of batter into the skillet and tilt the skillet in a circular motion so that the batter spreads over a large area. Cook 1 to 2 minutes, until lightly brown.

3. Flip the crêpe and cook it another minute. Remove it from the pan, fill with your favorite fillings, and fold it into quarters or roll it. For crêpes with sweet fillings, dust very lightly with confectioners' sugar if desired.

ARE WE THERE YET?
The Winding Road
Through the Threes

Between the ages of three and four, the pace of this journey may appear to slow down. Everything seems to be coming together for raising a budding foodie—a child's gross motor, fine motor, and oral motor skills are now well developed and her cognitive skills are becoming more refined, making it fun to really start "exploring" food. It's the perfect time to reflect on what strategies have brought us to this point. Let's continue to utilize what works, but we will adjust it just a bit for the older child.

TYPICAL MOTOR SKILL DEVELOPMENT
IN A NUTSHELL

During your child's third year, you'll notice that he is moving and exploring his world with three-year-old precision. He has established the gross motor stability to support the fine motor skills necessary for eating a variety of foods. In many ways, he's a mini-adult, including when it comes to eating. He can chew most foods, although some textures may be challenging if he has not had enough practice over time. Thanks to improved dexterity, during this year he will be able to use age-appropriate scissors and screw and unscrew jar lids. He is more precise as he helps you in the kitchen, layering wet lasagna noodles with spoonfuls of fillings, pouring liquids to the very top of the measuring cup without spilling, or using child-safe knives to help chop vegetables for the salad. It's almost bittersweet—he has come a long way in three short years!

Cognitive Skills Related to Feeding

In 2013, we teamed up to create "Doctor Yum's Preschool Food Adventure," a nutrition curriculum designed to teach preschoolers how to explore and enjoy healthy whole foods. Every month the curriculum features a new fruit or vegetable, which children explore with all of their senses. They also make a delicious snack using cooking skills they practice as they prepare. Your three-year-old can identify and name familiar colors and follow three-step directions with ease, such as, "Take the green peppers and mix them with the yellow peppers, then pour the mix in the pan." He can sort ingredients by size or shape and begin to count when asked to "find four big strawberries." He understands the concepts of same versus different, and uses comparison skills, such as, "It feels a lot like a crunchy apple in your mouth, but it tastes milder and it's called jicama."

Your child is primed for more educational experiences around food. Over the next year, your child's natural curiosity will prime the pump—it's time to learn about gardening and get our hands dirty! It's time to learn about kitchen science, like scrambling, boiling, and frying an egg. It's time to learn the basics of nutrition, and he's beginning to connect healthy food as fuel for our bodies. That curiosity will become obvious to you because you'll hear a barrage of "Why?" every single day. "Why does an egg get hard when you boil it, Mommy?" or "Daddy, why do potatoes grow underground but tomatoes don't?" The winding road through the threes opens up to a world of learning about food, and it promises to be memorable for both of you.

TOOLS FOR LITTLE CHEFS

Here are some tools that your three-year-old may use to help you in the kitchen:

Apron
Cutting mat (grippy on one side)
Kid-safe knives
Measuring spoons and cups (dry and liquid)
Mixing spoons
Salad spinner
Whisk

Lessons for Little Chefs

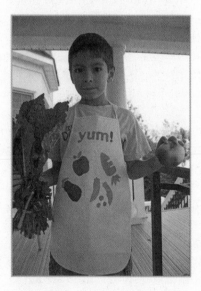

Three-year-olds are now able to get some cooking skills under their belts. First thing, they must look the part. In the Doctor Yum kitchen, kids are offered aprons that have stenciled fruits and veggies and the word "Yum" emblazoned across the front. You can make these easily at home. Craft stores are a perfect place to find plain canvas aprons in a small size. Get some fabric paint, stencils, and painting sponges to decorate the front. Your three-year-old will feel like a special chef when she wears her apron and will feel proud that she made it herself.

Introduce hand washing as the very first step in your cooking routine, and explain why it's important both before and after cooking. Now that your child is aproned, clean, and ready to go, position her in a safe place so that she is comfortable in helping with tasks. The Learning Tower is a safe platform that can bring your child to counter height, making it easier for her to participate and see what you're doing. The kitchen table is another place where it may be easy for your three-year-old to cook if you don't own a Learning Tower.

In the Doctor Yum classes and preschool curriculum, we introduce basic knife skills at ages three to four. Knife safety is stressed: We remind kids to put the knife flat on the table when it is not in use, and if they are carrying a knife to walk with the blade pointing down. It's important to offer them very safe knives to use, but also ones that can actually cut. Our favorite knife is the "Dog Knife" from the Swiss company Kuhn Rikon. These are sized for small hands, adorable, and easy to use. They are also very effective in cutting but, surprisingly, are not too sharp for new little chefs. We also show kids how to use the knife by holding it close to the blade and using the opposite hand to hold the food with a "cat claw" position so that they don't cut their fingers. At first, give them things to cut that are soft, like mushrooms, and precut certain round foods so that they can be placed flat on a cutting mat. Make sure you cut on a mat that is grippy on one side so that it does not slide easily.

There are plenty of tools like whisks, mixing spoons, and spatulas that are available in kid-friendly sizes and may be easier for your child to use than adult-sized utensils. One of preschoolers' favorite activities is to use a salad spinner to spin greens dry. This is one of those activities that will build familiarity with green leafy vegetables as they push the button on the spinner.

Let your little one measure ingredients with you and show them the cups used for wet and dry ingredients. Introduce basic measuring units like "teaspoon" and "tablespoon," and which is bigger. Continue to encourage cleanup skills by showing kids how to properly tidy up their workspace. Bring your Learning Tower or step stool up to the sink for washing pots, pans, and little hands.

MANAGING MEALTIME BEHAVIORS

- "But I don't like avocado anymore." When interest in healthy staples wanes
- Just eat already! Kids who eat too slowly
- "But now I really am hungry!" Kids who want to eat immediately after meals are over
- "I only want to eat what's on your plate."
- The roaming child: How to teach kids to stay at the table

It's been an interesting trek so far and the "threes" are the perfect time to take stock of what's working and what's not. Often, new undesirable behaviors can be addressed by reintroducing previous strategies or by fine-tuning them just a bit.

When Interest in a Healthy Staple Wanes

While your three-year-old may not refuse a food as strongly as she once did, she may become less than enthusiastic about a nutritious food she once craved. We all experience this when we enjoy a favorite food a little too often. We lose interest in it over time. The key is to take a short break from it (perhaps two weeks) and then reintroduce it in a new way. For example, let's say your child no longer wants to eat avocado.

Avocado is one of the healthiest foods, so it would be a shame for your child to skip it. It's loaded with good-for-you monounsaturated fat, it's higher in potassium than even a banana, and has lots of vitamins and protein. Plus, avocados are packed with fiber—eleven grams to be exact. That's about half of the fiber your three-year-old needs each day.

Here are six ways to serve this nutritious fruit (did you know it was a fruit and not a vegetable?) to arouse their curiosity once again:

1. Give your child a melon baller and a half of an avocado. How many scoops does it take to get to the empty shell?

2. Give him a plastic knife to crosshatch the avocado half. Afterward, show him how to use a large spoon to scoop out all the "puzzle pieces."

3. Avocado in a smoothie makes it ultra smooth and creamy.

4. In a powerful blender, avocado can become as fluffy as mousse. Add fruit to make "green pudding" or some cocoa powder and sweetener to make instant chocolate mousse.

5. If your family enjoys homemade guacamole, make your child the Guacamole Master! The repeated exposure to the chopped onions and tomatoes (or whatever you like to throw in there) plus tearing the cilantro as he makes the dip for the family can only help him see avocado in a whole new light.

6. Show your child how to smash a piece of avocado on a plate using his fork. Now, show her how to lightly sprinkle one of three different seasonings on different sections of the avocado. Taste test: Which seasoning does she like best? It's a terrific opportunity to tune in to her changing flavor preferences and incorporate those same flavors into new foods.

Our point is to change it up! Get creative and get your child involved in the process. Keep exposing him periodically to the food in fun and interactive ways to reignite his interest.

Coach Mel's Tip: Taste with Your Fingers

Tasting by dipping your finger into your own portion allows the brain to experience the food via the nerves on the fingertip first. Plus, when we put our finger on our tongue, we get proprioceptive feedback through the muscles and joints in our fingers as well as our tongues. Be sure to add a loud *pop!* with your lips in the process. This provides even more signals to the brain while helping to decrease gagging due to the increased input. Besides, it's just plain fun!

Dr. Yum's Tip: Be Sure to Feed Your Child These Five Nutrients

Jill Castle and Maryann Jacobsen, registered dietitians and authors who write about childhood nutrition, discuss the "fearless five nutrients" in their book *Fearless Feeding.* Castle and Jacobsen report that these five nutrients are critical for your child's growth: calcium, vitamin D, potassium, iron, and fiber.[68] Healthy staples for most of these nutrients include dairy products, fortified orange juice, spinach, almonds, and seeds, such as hemp or chia seeds.

When Kids Eat Too Slowly

While we applaud anyone who takes their time to enjoy a meal, some children are so talkative and social that they don't always get the full nutritional benefit of a mealtime. Here are three tips for speeding things up:

1. Set a timer away from the table for fifteen minutes: The purpose is to signal that the next activity is about to start. When the timer goes off, casually say, "It's not time yet, but soon we'll be doing (fill in activity here)." Because it takes about twenty minutes for the stomach to alert the brain that it is full, giving a gentle cue before that helps kids tune into the feeling of hunger.

2. The five-minute flag: When you suspect that mealtime is winding down, but he's been too chatty to judge that on his own, pull out the five-minute flag. This can be constructed out of anything—even a paper cup turned upside-down with a homemade flagpole (e.g., a straw or skewer) sticking out of it. Add a paper flag to the pole that says "EAT." Coach Mel likes to take a silly picture of her clients eating something yummy and put it on the flag. Teach your child that when the flag appears, it means "no talking, just eating" and model that. He might try to engage you during those five minutes, but don't give in. Just keep eating at a reasonable pace, enjoying your meal and don't respond except to occasionally whisper, "No talking, just eating." This strategy helps kids learn to focus on eating for just a short time—enough to eat a bit more if they feel hungry. Don't worry if he doesn't eat—it's not your responsibility to *make* your child eat. It's your job to help him learn to focus on the feeling of hunger and satisfy that need on his own. Social butterflies sometimes have a hard time with that, because they are so intent on chatting.

3. Teach "fast" and "slow": Sometimes three-year-olds just don't have a sound understanding of what slow, fast, and speeds in between truly mean. Be sure to teach these concepts throughout the day. Model them occasionally in real-life situations, including mealtimes: "Oh, I was so busy talking that I ate my soup too slowly. Now it's cold and I like to eat it warm."

It's not unusual for the very slow eater to be hungry again shortly after a mealtime. That can be frustrating for parents, but it's also the perfect learning opportunity for kids.

When Kids Declare, "I'm Hungry!" Right After Meals

Remember, we are teaching children to be responsible for putting healthy foods in their growing bodies, and that may mean experiencing hunger until the next meal or snack time. When a child dawdles or chooses not to eat during a meal, that's an opportunity for her to learn to tune in to what her body is telling her. A child who declares, "I'm hungry," right after twenty minutes at the table probably *was* hungry at the table. She either didn't tune in to that feeling, or she chose not to eat what was offered. If she is still feeling those pangs after the meal, that's OK. Be careful not to say, "Well you should have eaten at lunch!" Instead, parent consistently by simply saying, "We'll have a snack in two hours; that's after we go to the park." State the fact and move on. Don't get pulled into any drama. Your child is being reminded that there are growing times and eating times, as described in chapter 5 (page 99).

When Kids Say, "I don't want what's on my plate, Mommy, I want YOURS."

Turning three can be an emotional time for children. Their whole world changes as they transition to preschool, are introduced to structured community sports like T-ball and tot soccer, and encounter new sights and sounds at every turn. It can be an insecure time and can bring about behaviors like clinginess and wanting anything that connects them to Mom or Dad. That includes what's on your plate, even when the same food is on theirs. The key here is to establish some boundaries and parent consistently. Two responses you can implement include: "You can pick one thing off my plate and I'll give you one bite; that's the rule," and "We only eat what's on our own plates. You can have more afterward if you like."

When Kids Wander from the Table

By the time your child has turned three, he likely has the fine motor skills to unbuckle the safety belt on his feeding chair. This newfound independence is quite empowering and he may spontaneously leave the table before family dinnertime is over. To teach a child that mealtimes are an event shared with the entire family, regardless of whether he eats or not, try the following six strategies:

1. Keep a regular mealtime schedule with no grazing. Preschools use this strategy by posting a picture schedule on the bulletin board in the classroom. Help your child understand the daily schedule so that he anticipates the next event, including mealtimes.

2. Mark the beginning and the end of a meal with a song, a prayer, or a ritual that is special to your family. Kids benefit from structure and knowing what is about to happen and, likewise, when the meal is over. Thus, be sure to mark the *end* of the meal by having even the youngest kids take their plates to the kitchen counter or sink when they are done eating. If your child declares that he is done and gets down from the table, remind him to take his plate to the counter. Whatever he does away from the table, try to give him very little attention. If he returns to the table, welcome him back with, "Oh, we were just talking about that funny thing that happened at preschool today!" or something similar to bring him into conversation. By engaging him at the table, you are reinforcing the behavior of being at the table. If he asks for something to eat, be casual and state the fact: "Oh sweetie, you took your plate to the counter, showing me that you were done eating. We'll have snack in a few hours." Now, engage him again about something totally different than food. "You were so silly at preschool today! Tell Daddy how you made everyone laugh with your monkey impressions! Daddy loves monkeys. . . ." If he has a meltdown, address the meltdown as you would at any other time, but don't respond with offering him anything off your plate or returning his plate to the table.[69]

3. Even if your child requires a liquid calorie supplement, serve filling drinks, including milk, at the end of the meal and limit to four ounces with each meal for kids ages four and up. By now, your child is getting daily calcium from other sources, including a variety of dairy products and/or various greens, and even four ounces of milk three times per day meets almost half of his daily requirement. Calcium is an important nutrient, but it's easy to over-rely on glasses of milk, which in turn can stop appetite in its tracks.

4. Revisit proper positioning. As kids grow, it's tempting to let them kneel on an adult chair or sit in a chair that's just a bit too big for them. Like any tabletop activity, having a good, supportive chair makes the time at the table much more enjoyable and you're likely to stay at the table longer. Please refer to chapter 5 (page 72) for a review of ideal seating options for kids.

5. Avoid distractions while eating, both at and away from the table. Is the TV on in the next room? Are your cell phones sitting on the dinner table? A small toy at the table that facilitates parent-child interaction is fine, but mindless distractions don't allow for learning to engage with others at the table.[70]

6. It's OK to allow one trip to the bathroom. It's not unusual for young children (and some adults) to have the urge to have a bowel movement as the stomach fills during a meal. This is due to the gastrocolic reflex, most obvious in infants when they make a dirty diaper after a feeding, yet still present as kids grow. Although we gain more control over it with time, it's permissible to allow one trip to the bathroom in the midst of a meal. Try to be very matter-of-fact about it and don't allow any playtime in the trip to and from the bathroom. Upon returning to the table together, let the fun begin again.[71]

When shaping a child's behavior, it's all about what you respond to and being consistent with that response. It takes time. In fact, if consistency did not take time, it wouldn't meet the definition of "consistent," which means "steady continuity." A behavior has to receive reinforcement over time to eventually become habit.

EXPLORING FOOD AWAY FROM MEALTIMES

- Food discovery away from mealtimes: It's essential!
- Breakfast boosts brainpower.
- When there are medical factors: Kids who must eat.
- Parenting styles: Which passport stamps work for you?

There are times to expose kids to food away from a meal—and it's all about keeping it fun. Let's revisit a previous strategy but tweak it just a bit for the three-year-olds' level of fine motor and cognitive skills. As we've discussed, food exploration apart from meals is crucial for engaging kids in all aspects of food. The more they interact with the food, the more likely they are to try it eventually. Now that your three-year-old has the attention and dexterity to create crafts with you, try these ideas with your young artist:

Beet Stamping: Beets come in all sorts of colors, from yellow to purple to red. Stamping is simple: Just slice off the end of the beet for your child, leaving the leafy green part to use as a handle. For the more hesitant eater, give him a paintbrush to paint the flat side with water and then stamp onto craft paper. For the more adventurous, let him lick his beet to get it wet and then stamp! Create cut-outs in the beets with a paring knife, like a smiley face or a fun design.

Celery Stamping: There are many different designs you can create with celery stamps. First, cut off all the stalks about four inches from the base. Keep the leaves on the stalks. If you dip the flat side of the base in homemade edible paint (see next item), you'll have a perfect imprint of a rose. You can also tie any combination of stalks together to create flowers of different shapes. As you and your child are bundling stalks, talk about the properties of celery. Pull some of the strings down the sides and use those to make wisps of grass in your picture. Use the leaves as paintbrushes—let your imagination take over!

Stamping and painting is possible with any vegetable. Experiment with your child. It's fun to say, "I've never tried this—what do you think we can make with jicama? How about with cauliflower?" It's the perfect way to raise interest again while shopping in the produce aisle together: "Ooooh, what kind of picture do you think we could make with a kohlrabi?"

Edible Paint Recipes: Using a muffin tin, you and your child can mix up the following variations of edible paint. Just choose a base, add color from *real* food, and thin if necessary with a touch of water.

BASE	REAL FOOD COLORING	MAKES THIS COLOR
Plain or vanilla yogurt—dairy or nondairy versions	Juice from mashed beets—use a variety of colors—or from canned beets	Red, yellow, orange, or purple
Homemade whipped cream	Carrots pulverized in a food processor or blender, or bottled carrot juice	Orange, unless using colored carrots like purple
Ripe avocado whipped in the blender	Spinach pulverized in a food processor or blender	Green

Dr. Yum's Tip:
Read Labels to Avoid Food Dyes

If you start to offer more store-bought foods without paying attention to labels, it can be easy for additives and artificial colors to make their way into your child's diet. In a recent review of the past three decades of research on food dyes, it was found that in a subset of children there are significant changes in attention span and concentration when kids ingest 100 mg of food dye daily,[72] the same amount found in 2 cups of macaroni and cheese, 8 ounces of an orange soft drink, and a small bag of Skittles. Another recent study demonstrated how prevalent food dyes are in many common foods offered to children and quantified how much dye is contained in those foods. Add up drinks and candies with food dyes to other common foods like boxed mac and cheese, crackers, and breakfast cereals, and it is easy to imagine how many kids in America can top 100 mg of food dye daily.[73] If you're trying to avoid food dyes, then make sure to read labels carefully and make homemade versions of store-bought favorites.

Breakfast: Thinking Outside the Cereal Box

Breakfast is one meal that really is important. Children should start off the day with a nutritious meal that is also going to fuel them all morning. Research has demonstrated that preschool children who ate breakfast on a regular basis didn't just do better in school than kids who "sometimes" had breakfast, they did significantly better on IQ tests. The relationship between breakfast and test scores was even adjusted for "gender, current living location, parental education, and occupation" to ensure that it was the all-important morning meal that set the child up for a successful day of learning and brain development.[74]

Many average breakfasts are carbohydrate-heavy with a lot of simple sugars. When insulin spikes in response to all the carbs, it can leave kids hungry before their next meal. Also, many typical breakfasts do not include fruits or vegetables. Most kids in America do not get the recommended amount of fruits and vegetables in a day, and a breakfast that does not include produce is a missed opportunity to meet that important goal. For an optimal breakfast, make sure to include some protein, which will help kids maintain energy throughout the morning. Also, use breakfast to get in a serving of fruits and veggies. Throw some berries on your child's oatmeal or offer sliced mango as a side. In short, try these five tips for helping morning mealtimes go well:

1. Wake up hungry: Keep bedtime snacks light so that kids wake up ready to eat a healthy breakfast.

2. Plan ahead: Prep breakfast the night before. Energy bites or soaked oats are just two options that are as convenient as cereal.

3. Remember produce: Add one of our rainbow smoothies to your favorite breakfast. Also, don't miss the Friteeni Frittatas recipe at the end of this chapter—it's a super-easy recipe for making ahead and swiftly reheating the next morning. Now you've included that vital serving of vegetables.

4. Protein power! Add a punch of protein to keep energy up all morning. Even a half of a banana topped with nut butter can make all the difference.

5. Don't be a breakfast boss: Try not to start your child's day with a commanding tone or insist that kids eat breakfast. With time, the three strategies noted above will work, so parent patiently and consistently. If you tend to be the boss of breakfast, try to let that go.

Weekend mornings are such a precious time for families. For Dr. Yum, it meant making crêpes with melted butter and sugar or fresh fruit. When Coach Mel was a little girl, it was often pancakes or buying a donut after Sunday services in the church basement. We all have our family traditions, and why not switch it up every once in a while with a breakfast activity that gets your kids thinking about new types of breakfast foods? One of our favorites is building kebabs by alternating fruit chunks, pieces of healthy muffins, or a few energy bites (see recipe chart). You and your kids can make your own favorite versions by combining a variety of dried fruits, nuts, and more—the combinations just might be endless! Plus, they're not just a breakfast food: Energy bites keep for several days in the refrigerator and make a delicious addition to lunches or a quick after-school snack. Just follow these directions:

How to Make Energy Bites

1: Binder	2: Dried Fruit	3: Protein Puree	4: Sweetener	5: Nuts	6: Optional Power Boost	7: Roll balls in . . .
1 cup	1/2 cup	1/4 cup	1/4 cup or less	1/2 cup or less	1 to 2 tablespoons	
dry oatmeal, ground or whole	chopped dates	nut butter	honey	coarsely chopped walnuts	ground flax seeds	coconut
finely chopped raw cashews	chopped dried cherries	seed butter	agave nectar	coarsely chopped pecans	whole hemp	raw cacao powder
finely chopped raw almonds	chopped dried apricots	baked squash puree	coconut sugar	sunflower seeds, shelled	chia seeds	dusting of cinnamon and superfine sugar

1: Binder	2: Dried Fruit	3: Protein Puree	4: Sweetener	5: Nuts	6: Optional Power Boost	7: Roll balls in...
whole grain cereal of your choice, smashed	chopped dried apples or a mix of dried fruits	pumpkin puree	maple syrup	coarsely chopped peanuts	whole pumpkin seeds (pepitas)	1/2 cup mini chocolate chips or cacao nibs

Using a food processor, simply pulse and combine one item from column one and column two. Stir in the puree from column three, then drizzle in the sweetener from column four, being careful not to make the mixture too sticky. Now, transfer the mixture to a bowl to add more ingredients. Add just enough chopped nuts or seeds from column five to make the dough malleable and easy to roll into balls about the size of a ping-pong ball. Sprinkle in the power boosts from column six for an optional punch of omega-3 fatty acids, omega-6 fatty acids, and protein. Finally, roll the balls in something yummy from column seven. Refrigerate until ready to serve. How many different variations can you make?

Pumpkin Pepita Bites: Add 1 teaspoon cinnamon, ⅛ teaspoon ground nutmeg, and ½ teaspoon ground ginger to pumpkin puree. Mix as directed these ingredients from the following columns: 1. Oats, 2. Dates, 3. Pumpkin puree with spices, 4. Honey, 5. Nuts or seeds, 6. Power boost, and 7. Roll in pepitas.

Salted Chocolate Bites: Mix as directed these ingredients from the following columns: 1. Binder of your choice, 2. Cherries, 3. Nut butter or seed butter, 4. Sweetener of your choice plus 1 teaspoon vanilla and 1 teaspoon raw cacao powder, 5. Nuts or seeds (cashews are ideal!), 6. Power boost of your choice, and 7. Roll in cacao and/or chocolate chips. After rolling, sprinkle just the tops of balls with a dash of sea salt—pink Himalayan salt is extra pretty on these!

Apple-Blueberry Surprise: Use dried apples and blueberries from column two and your favorite combination of ingredients from the other columns in the chart. With a toothpick, push a dried cranberry, a big chocolate chip, or a toasted pecan into the center to create a yummy surprise.

Chocolate-Ginger-Snap Bites: Mix as directed these ingredients from the following columns: 1. Almonds, 2. Dates and cherries, 3. Nut or seed butter, 4. Any sweetener, plus ½ teaspoon grated ginger, 5. Nuts or seeds, 6. Power boost, and 7. Roll in chocolate chips.

• •

ELIZABETH'S STORY:
A Family Learns to Relax at the Dinner Table

One of the aspects of her job that Coach Mel enjoys most is working with families in their homes. One particular family was memorable because both parents were security guards, and they seemed to bring an element of their jobs to the family dinner table. They contacted Mel because their preschooler, Elizabeth, wasn't gaining weight and was a "very picky eater." Upon arriving at the home, Coach Mel was delighted to see both parents completely engaged with their little girl, all three laughing and playing together on the living room floor.[75]

Interestingly, the atmosphere shifted the moment everyone sat down at the table. There was practically no conversation except to announce what was for dinner and how much the little girl was expected to eat. "Remember to eat all your corn, Elizabeth," her father stated. The parents watched over her vigilantly and occasionally reminded her to "keep eating." When the couple had finished their meal, and Elizabeth was staring at her not-so-empty plate, her father reprimanded her for "not eating her corn . . . again." Both parents felt the need to set stringent eating rules, enforce them, and remind Elizabeth if she did not follow dinnertime guidelines. Clearly, their concern for her growth and nutrition were in the forefront of their minds, but why did they feel this authoritarian approach would be helpful? What happened to those parents joyfully interacting with their little girl in the living room?

Parenting styles evolve over time and are dependent on not only the child's temperament, but the parent's personalities as well. We've all learned certain parenting practices from the way we were raised and adjust those over time as our relationships with our own children change. It turns out that both parents had grown up in very commanding households. Their strict nature at the dinner table (and the same attitude needed in their jobs) was exactly how they were raised years ago. "It must be the right thing to do," they reasoned, because "they ate just fine" and had no memories of mealtimes being a struggle while growing up. Still, these parents recognized that the watchdog approach wasn't a good fit with their daughter's hesitant eating style. For the naturally adventurous eater, this may be because there really is nothing to enforce if the child is an eager eater anyway. But as we've discussed thus far, there is so much more to raising adventurous eaters. It's about the whole child.[76]

Diana Baumrind, a clinical and developmental psychologist, identified at least three different types of parenting styles: authoritarian, authoritative, and permissive.[77] Many parents shift in style according to specific events or the environment, being more permissive in certain settings and stricter in others. This particular family adopted stricter rules with high expectations for eating vegetables and finishing what was served, requiring young Elizabeth to accept their rules without discussion. Authoritarian parents leave a child with very little room for independent decision making and responding to internal cues (e.g., lack of hunger) to drive personal behavior (e.g., eating corn).[78]

While the authoritarian style lies at one end of Baumrind's parenting spectrum, the permissive parent (otherwise known as the child's best friend) lies at the other. Permissive parents set very few limits. As it relates to feeding, permissive parents let kids graze on whatever the kids want to eat throughout the day. While nurturing and loving, these parents avoid conflict with their kids and are comfortable indulging the child's whims, as long as their kiddo is happy. They become short-order cooks, justifying their own behavior by saying, "Just make her pasta again—at least she'll eat that."[79]

In the middle of the spectrum lies authoritative parenting, characterized by parents who set safe boundaries for their kids while providing opportunities for their children to make autonomous decisions. This parent prepares healthy meals for children, presents the food in a relaxed manner, and allows the child to listen to internal cues to determine how much they need to eat. Parents provide structure and opportunities to explore food while modeling healthy eating.[80] Coach Mel helped Elizabeth's parents to bring their naturally authoritative parenting style (demonstrated in other parts of the day) to the family dinner table and let go of being the food police.

Although Baumrind's model was established back in the sixties and has certainly elicited discussions on its pros and cons, for the sake of reflection it's helpful to have guidelines. We like to use these seven parenting concepts that consider the whole child: parenting proactively and with patience, consistency, bravery, compassion, mindfulness, and above all else, joy. Whatever model you use, be sure to reflect on what's working and what's not, and adjust accordingly.

• •

When Kids Must Eat

When a child has certain medical diagnoses, like type 1 diabetes or failure to thrive, parents feel pressure to ensure that their child consumes enough calories. Type 1 diabetes (previously termed "juvenile diabetes") is a condition that often presents in childhood. In this condition, pancreatic islet cells that produce the hormone insulin are destroyed by the child's own immune system, leaving their body unable to regulate blood sugar. Insulin therefore has to be administered to children via injections throughout the day or by an insulin pump. Food intake needs to be carefully regulated along with the administration of insulin so the blood sugar stays in a safe range.

Other diagnoses that would make it important for children to eat include "underweight" or "failure to thrive." Underweight is a term pediatricians use to describe children whose weight falls below the fifth percentile. On its own, underweight may not be concerning to your pediatrician, especially if your child is growing parallel to a standard growth curve, and if many other family members tend to be small. On the other hand, failure to thrive refers to children whose growth is not following the expected rate and their weight may be dropping. There are literally hundreds of conditions that could cause a child to not achieve an ideal growth velocity, and often your team of health care providers will focus on making sure the child eats an ideal amount of calories to reverse the trend. This medical diagnosis can be frightening to parents and may force them to focus more than ever on how much their child is eating. With any of these diagnoses, the added pressure can create secondary behavioral issues and some very stressful mealtimes for both the child and the parents.

 Dr. Yum's Tip: "Failure to Thrive" Doesn't Mean You're Failing

The diagnosis of failure to thrive is one that can feel defeating for many parents, but despite the terminology, it has nothing to do with failing. It simply is a diagnosis that must be used so that your baby can receive the help she needs to get on track. The focus is on growth or thriving. A baby may need certain tests, referrals to specialists, a special diet, or other services that will require that diagnosis in order for those steps to occur.

When a child must eat, a registered dietitian will offer tips for boosting calories per bite, plus you may want to implement some of the strategies we've noted earlier in this chapter. Healthy calorie boosters include coconut oil, avocado, bananas, and nuts or seeds (if no allergies are present). Some liquid supplements provide additional calories, too. One of our favorite prepackaged nutritional shakes is from Orgain Healthy Kids. Smoothies are another way to provide healthy, nutritious, and calorie-packed snacks. If your child has type 1 diabetes, be sure to balance the carbohydrates as directed by your child's health practitioner. For extra calories that aren't too filling, consider hemp seeds, chia seeds, frozen bananas, whole milk yogurts, and/or some coconut oil for added sweetness. How about some sunflower butter? Toss in a handful of spinach or kale, too—it will disappear like magic if the smoothie has a dark-colored berry in the mix.

A RAINBOW OF SMOOTHIES*	Red: Sweetheart Smoothie	Orange: Scarecrow Smoothie
	1 cup strawberries 1 cup raspberries 1 banana 1 cup red grapes 1 cup chopped kale ice	2 cups green grapes 1 orange 1 sweet potato, cooked and cooled ½ cup cranberries 2 dates, pitted ½ teaspoon grated ginger ice
Yellow: Sunshine Smoothie	Green: Green Dragon Smoothie	Blue: Indi-GO Smoothie
1 banana 1 mango, peeled and diced 2 slices pineapple squeeze of lime juice ice	1 cup green grapes 2 slices pineapple ½ banana 1 orange ½ lime wedge with skin ice ½ teaspoon ginger, grated	1 medium banana 1 to 2 cups red grapes 1 cup blueberries 1 cup chopped kale ½ carrot ice

*Add-ins to pack your smoothie with healthy calories: almond butter, almond milk, avocado, chia seeds, coconut milk, coconut oil, flax meal, full-fat plain Greek yogurt, oatmeal, soaked raw cashews, or sunflower butter, just to name a few.

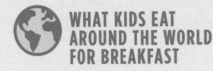

WHAT KIDS EAT AROUND THE WORLD FOR BREAKFAST

In many parts of the world, breakfast is a well-rounded meal with protein, fruits, and vegetables and may resemble lunch or dinner more than the sweet breakfast that we know. Here are two examples of breakfast in other parts of the world.

In Vietnam, breakfast may consist of savory rice porridge, very similar to Chinese congee. It is eaten sometimes just plain or topped with some boiled chicken, scallions, and cilantro. Sometimes this dish may be topped with pickled cucumbers or bamboo shoots, or sautéed greens like spinach. *Pho* is a traditional rice noodle soup with a beef or chicken broth and is served with garnishes like Thai basil, cilantro, bean sprouts, and lime wedges. This popular dish is served at any time of day, including breakfast.

In Egypt, *ful medames* (stewed fava beans) are a breakfast staple and may be served with an egg and pita bread. Fava beans may be cooked in oil with tomato, parsley, garlic, and lemon juice and spiced with cumin or tahini. This breakfast is packed with protein and fiber and is a great start to the day!

Friteeni Frittatas

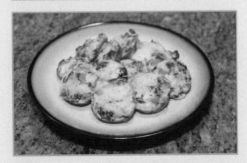

Dr. Yum loves to teach kids how to make a healthy breakfast in her popular "Doctor Yum's Pajama Party" class. Kids come dressed in their coziest pajamas to learn how to make some of her breakfast recipes, and this one is always a favorite. A frittata is a baked omelet and is a great way to introduce your favorite veggies into breakfast. This teeny, tiny version is made in muffin cups, making them adorable and attractive to kids. Serve these with sides like fruit, whole grain bread, or steel-cut oatmeal. The eggs are packed with protein, which means your little ones will stay full all morning. The frittatas store and reheat well for dinner or breakfast the next day, too.

Makes 24 mini-frittatas

8 large eggs
¼ to ⅓ cup milk
salt
1 tablespoon olive oil, plus more for oiling the pan
1 onion, finely diced
1 large sweet potato, peeled and finely diced
    (about 2 cups)
3 cups thinly sliced Swiss chard
    (spinach or kale can also be substituted)
1 teaspoon finely chopped fresh rosemary
ground pepper
½ cup grated Parmesan cheese

1. Preheat the oven to 375°F. Beat the eggs, milk, and a dash of salt in a medium bowl and set aside. Lightly coat two muffin tins with olive oil using a paper towel.

2. Heat 1 tablespoon olive oil in a large skillet over medium heat. Cook the onions 2 to 3 minutes, until slightly soft. Add the sweet potatoes and cook about 4 to 6 minutes, until soft. Add the Swiss chard and rosemary and cook other 4 minutes or so, until the greens are wilted. Season with salt and pepper.

3. Fill each muffin cup with about a tablespoon of cooked vegetables. Spoon 1 to 2 tablespoons of egg mixture into each cup so that the vegetables are nearly covered.

4. Bake about 10 to 12 minutes. Remove the tins and sprinkle a pinch of Parmesan cheese on each little frittata. Return the tins to the oven for another 5 minutes, or until the eggs are cooked through (watch carefully so they don't brown too much). Remove each frittata with a silicone spatula and serve warm.

Coach Mel's Tip: Wide Straws = More Calories with Each Swallow

When you need to add calories to your child's daily intake, offer a wide straw with smoothies. For kids who have age-appropriate oral motor skills, a wider straw delivers more smoothie into the mouth and slightly more calories with each swallow. As long as solid foods are a part of daily mealtimes, periodically drinking healthy calories is an easy way of helping a child get extra nutrition without adding stress to the mix, too.

What an exciting journey so far! You and your child have had so many positive food experiences. Congratulate yourself for all the hard work you have put in. It's paying off as we round the corner to age four. You have set the stage for the next leg of your journey when the outside world may challenge the healthy habits you have established.

UNEXPECTED GUESTS, AKA THE INFLUENCE OF THE OUTSIDE WORLD
Ages Four to Six

· ·

The ages of four to six are when your child becomes more aware of his external environment. He is now going to school regularly, spending more time with peers on some days than he will with his family. He will also develop reasoning skills that can help him understand how his independent choices have consequences. Now is the time to show him that the adventurous eating style you have taught him has a reason and a purpose. You also want to build on that foundation by using the environment as a canvas for new lessons about food. The grocery store, the garden, and the sports field are all places you can apply healthy eating, reinforcing what you have taught him already and keeping him on the right track—despite unhealthy food choices he may encounter at every turn. Know that you may pick up some unexpected guests on the road ahead, but bringing them into your culture of wellness makes for the most successful journey possible.

TYPICAL MOTOR SKILL DEVELOPMENT IN A NUTSHELL

Four- to six-year-olds now have a foundation of developmental skills but are still flying through new ones every day. From a gross motor standpoint, they have developed more balance and should be able to stand on one foot for a few seconds. They may learn to do a somersault or hop on one foot and can learn to skip with some practice. As they are stronger now, they can take on more tasks in the kitchen like passing serving bowls around or setting a table. Their fine motor skills are allowing them to explore art further, like drawing and copying more complex shapes. This skill helps them to learn to copy letters and write their own names, and also explore art with food, like decorating a gingerbread house or arranging fruit on a plate. These fine motor skills will teach them to be more independent in dressing and caring for themselves and also in completing tasks in the kitchen.

Cognitive Skills Related to Feeding

Kids at this age are sophisticated little students. Their vocabulary is becoming more colorful as they use many more descriptive words to explain the world around them. This comes in handy when they are explaining the experience of trying new foods. They have a growing understanding of how they fit into a group and can follow more rules as this understanding (and patience) grows. They learn to take turns and share jobs in the kitchen with family members or in a cooking class. They can follow concepts of time, like how to read a clock, which can help when preparing recipes that need time to bake, simmer, rest, or rise before the next step. They are really ready to *understand* food and what it does for their bodies. They can also comprehend that learning to love new foods can take practice.

PROVIDING A FOOD EDUCATION

- How a garden can set the stage for healthy eating
- How kids can participate in shopping for food
- Food as part of their greater community

Your child is now able to start to understand the importance of food in daily life. In the hectic world we live in, it's easy to forget the value of feeding our bodies delicious and nutritious food. Take a minute to pause and think about that. This is the stage where you get to impart your family's food culture and how food choices impact not only the family, but also the community. Know that even if you as a parent did not grow up in a household that prioritized the quality and experience of food, you can build your own food culture with your growing family and increase your child's awareness.

Start a Garden and Show Your Child That Food Comes from the Earth

Up until this age, your child may not have had a complete understanding of where food comes from. But now your kids can learn that many foods come from the earth and that you can actually grow delicious food in your own backyard!

There are so many amazing reasons to start a garden with your child. Gardening is great exercise, and just like the food you grow, you and your kids can get the fresh air and sunshine you need. Kids can learn the valuable lessons of planning and executing a garden from start to finish. Also, for kids who are still exploring and trying new foods, garden-grown produce offers the tastiest and best chance for successful tasting. Dr. Yum's office has a garden out back, which serves as an outdoor waiting space and a place for her cooking students to explore growing food. One of her favorite things is to see her preschool students picking sun-ripened cherry tomatoes and eating them off the vines like it's the best treat they ever had! A review of school gardening studies showed that gardening is associated with improved science test scores and food behaviors.[81]

It's easy to see why, as starting a garden can spark an endless string of questions from your preschooler. Plan to answer questions about how plants breathe, get nutrients and water, and produce fruits and vegetables. There are tons of ways to expand on your garden experience, like finding coloring pages about plants, visiting a farm, or taking a trip to a botanical garden. At Dr. Yum's teaching garden some of preschoolers' favorite jobs are to water plants from the rain barrel and compost the scraps from the cooking lessons, both of which teach important lessons of sustainability.

There are many ways to start a garden, and you don't need a large outdoor space to do it. First, make sure that your child has appropriate garden tools, gloves, and footwear. Remember, getting messy is part of the fun of starting a garden! Lastly, decide on the type of garden that you and your child want to grow. Here are five easy ways that you can plant a garden with your kids:[82]

1. Plant right in the ground. Find a sunny spot in the yard where you can plant a small veggie patch. Typically a spot that gets at least six hours of sun is ideal. Make sure the soil is fertile and drains well. Use the help of local gardening supply shops to find products like compost to improve your soil.

2. Plant in existing landscaping. If your best sun is the front of your house, never fear! Edibles can be integrated with existing landscaping without looking messy or unstructured. If there is not a lot of space, consider using a pretty trellis or fencing to grow vegetables like cucumbers and squash vertically. Try using blueberry bushes, kale, thornless blackberries, and other edibles to replace some of the existing landscape. Kids will enjoy some of the fruits and veggies grown right in their own front yard!

3. Plant a raised bed garden. If your soil is poor and you don't feel like digging up your lawn, a raised garden is a great option for growing a lot of food in a small space. Many hardware stores sell inexpensive kits made of wood or plastic. Snap or nail the sides together, place in a sunny spot, fill with soil, and you're ready to go! *Square Foot Gardening* by Mel Bartholomew is a great resource that can get you started, and their website has even more resources to help you map out your garden. Small square-foot garden kits can be inexpensive and make great donations to a school so that students can learn to grow plants as a group.

4. Plant in containers. Don't have a backyard for growing? No problem! Edibles like tomatoes and herbs can easily be grown in containers filled with soil. This is a great way for kids to grow food without a lot of work for you. Kids love growing herbs like basil, thyme, oregano, and rosemary on a back porch in various pots. Let kids identify herbs by the shape of their leaves and their smell. Growing herbs saves a lot of money, too, as they can be harvested all summer long and even frozen for use in cold weather months.

5. Join a community garden. This is a fun way for kids to become part of a gardening community. Typically a small plot in a community garden can be rented for a small fee and used throughout the seasons to grow different types of edibles.

Once you have a plan for your garden, pick a few vegetables that are easy to grow. Zucchini, radishes, beans, tomatoes, lettuce, and other greens do not require a lot of work to maintain. Check online for planting times according to your growing zone. Greens like lettuce grow best in cooler weather like spring and fall, while tomatoes and squash are started in spring but thrive in warm weather.

Grocery Shopping Is an Education in Food Choices

Over the years, Dr. Yum has taught many grocery store classes to people who are looking for healthy ways to feed their families while saving money. She has observed, time and again, how young children are able to understand nutrition concepts and how easily they can be engaged in making healthy choices at the grocery store. One of things that she teaches families is to give the kids a simple task, like, "Find a cereal with less than five grams of sugar in a serving." She shows them where to find the sugar on the label and then watches while kids enthusiastically check cereal boxes up and down the aisle. When they realize their favorite cereals have too much sugar, they search for an acceptable substitute, saying, "Wow, we found one! This one only has two grams. Can we try it, Mom?" After one class, a mother reported that her seven-year-old son explained to his little brother over breakfast that they were going to try new cereals with less sugar. He told his brother that he could help him check the labels when they shopped next time, and showed him where the numbers could be found!

 Dr. Yum's Tip: Explain Food Choices to Your Kids While You Shop

When shopping with kids, take the time to explain the food choices you make. As they learn to read, show them food labels and explain how some ingredients can give their bodies energy while other ingredients, when eaten frequently, may make their body feel sick. Get them invested in making healthy choices so that food shopping becomes a more positive, team-building experience for your family. To make shopping more interesting, let your child pick a healthy recipe to shop for, challenge her to help you fill the cart with different colors of produce, or let her pick a new, interesting fruit or vegetable to try.

Shopping Locally

Farmers' markets are another great place to expand your child's food education. As with gardening, produce that is local will definitely taste better than the same items grown hundreds of miles away. As you become familiar with the farmers who sell at your market, they can be a great resource, letting you try new items that are in season and giving you preparation ideas. The farmers' market is where young foodies learn that a boxed tomato from a grocery store doesn't come close to the deliciousness of an heirloom tomato grown in their own county. This is where love affairs with local peaches, in-season strawberries, and cheese from grass-fed cows start. It's a wonderful thing to see your children pass up the bakery items at the farmers' market to find their favorite variety of locally grown apricots.

Also, shopping locally for food teaches kids important lessons about how taking time to pick out the best-tasting food really makes a difference. It shows them that there can be a deep and meaningful connection to the food they eat and that local, in-season food is better for the environment. It also starts the conversation about how supporting local farmers is important to sustaining their community.

Joining a CSA (community supported agriculture) by purchasing a share in a farm for a season is another great way to buy locally. Many farms offer this service, which can be a great value for families, too. By buying a share, you can enjoy local produce all season, and for young kids there is a lot of fun in being part of a CSA. Every week, you pick up a box of produce from the farm, and some of it may not be what you would not ordinarily buy. This arrangement provides kids many opportunities to taste new foods and for you family to try some new recipes.

NAVIGATING AND CHANGING THE FOOD CULTURE AROUND YOU

- How to get around the junk food everywhere
- How to make your kids savvy about food advertising
- How to make sports snacks healthier

Junk Food at the Grocery Store (and Everywhere Else You Go)

The food industry targets kids with clever marketing, advertising, and fancy packaging of highly processed foods made with artificial ingredients. We as parents can fight back by perfecting the skill of saying no at the grocery store. Saying no to a child can be difficult. It goes against our instinct to keep our children happy and comfortable. However, in some instances it is necessary, even though it may cause feelings of discomfort and frustration in our children. This paradox is one that we should embrace: Saying no can be the greatest show of love.

Let's face it. Grocery shopping with children is tough enough. The kids may be tired, hungry, and bored while we drag them down aisle after aisle. Now, add the temptation of highly attractive but unhealthy processed food, and it can be easy to break down and give in. Develop some ways of saying no to these requests, keeping your goal of healthy, educated eaters in mind. Saying no does not have to sting. It can be done with warmth, love, and compassion. Saying no may also create a teachable moment, in which kids can come away having learned a lesson about healthy eating.

First, put yourself in the position of a child. Children are bombarded by advertising and lured by smart, attractive packaging— often at their eye level. Grocery stores also are set up to tempt them into asking for unhealthy food. Children like what they see and do not know any better. They do not know that highly processed, colorful, fun-shaped foods with their artificial sweeteners, preservatives, and dyes can cause them a myriad of health issues later (or not so much later) in life. It's our job to say no and to protect them from the dangerous consequences of these artificial foods.

Junk food is not only at the grocery store. Having ground rules about where you buy food can help you avoid buying junk food where you shop for gas, fabric, sports gear, electronics, medications, and office supplies. All types of stores have realized that by putting junk food right at your child's eye level, they can increase sales. Keep to a consistent script: "We only buy food at the grocery store, and we have better choices at home to eat." Again, consistency is key to establishing the rule.

How to Fuel Your Young Athlete

Physical activity is so important, and many parents will sign up their kids for organized sports from a young age. Sports offer a chance for regular physical activity, socialization, and to get some fresh air after a long day at school. However, all too often we observe kids consuming unhealthy snacks as part of the sports experience. Well-meaning parents and coaches who want to fuel

A CLOSER LOOK:
Saying No

Here are some artful ways of saying no using all of the parenting principles and keeping your kids' health in mind:

1. Say "No" compassionately: Offer an alternative to a food they want. For instance, you might say, "Those cookies look nice, but I think I have a recipe for something almost like that, and it will be a lot healthier. Maybe we can make them together."

2. Say "No" mindfully: Provide an explanation and create a teachable moment. For instance, you might say, "No, I don't buy those kind of fruit snacks because they have dye in them that gives them bright colors. Some people can get really sick from those dyes. Can I show you on the label?" The child may then understand that the "no" comes with a good reason, and that you're looking out for them.

3. Say "No" proactively: Try to time your shopping after a meal. Hungry kids (and parents) are much more likely to give in to the pressures and temptations of unhealthy snack foods and treats while roaming the aisles. Be proactive and shop when tummies are already full.

4. Say "No" consistently: Lay ground rules early so you do not have to say no as much. For example, set a rule that you don't buy candy in checkout aisles. Once it's established, you won't have to battle at every grocery trip. At first it will take a lot of repetition: "Sorry, Mommy doesn't buy candy near the cash register." However, after several requests, they will get the message. Parenting consistently in those situations is tough (especially during a tantrum), but it only takes a few denials to get the rule established. It also only takes a few times of giving in to establish the consistent request for candy.

5. Say "No" joyfully: Celebrate with a small treat for cooperating at the grocery store. If buying a small non-food trinket every once in a while means you can get a cart full of healthy, whole foods,

then consider this an acceptable concession (and a small victory). Even more meaningful is offering special time with you or a privilege for being a good helper at the grocery store.

6. Say "No" bravely: Make a shopping list and don't be afraid to stick to it! Start off the shopping trip by laying down rules that you're buying only what's on the list and not much else. Making a list saves time (and money, too). Engage kids by asking them to find items on the list. For kids who aren't reading yet, make it extra fun for everyone by giving clues: "Find me a round fruit with skin you can peel off." You might be surprised how many different fruits they'll pick up and put in the grocery cart!

7. Say "No" patiently: Take the time to teach your kids how to spot unhealthy food. This works great for kids who are beginning to read and can be shown how to navigate a food label. Show them that the front of a package can paint a picture of a healthy choice while the nutritional information and ingredients on the back of the package can show the opposite. What are the first three ingredients? That tells you what's in *most* of that package. Have them weed out foods with high fructose corn syrup, food dyes, or other unhealthy ingredients. This way they will be keeping hundreds of processed foods out of your grocery cart.

and reward their team after a game choose snacks that they think their team will like. However, many of the foods and drinks provided are lower in nutrition and much higher in calories than what young athletes actually burn during their game. For instance, we observe young children being offered sports drinks, which can be a source of unnecessary calories and artificial ingredients. According to a clinical report by the American Academy of Pediatrics, regular consumption of sports drinks can contribute to overweight, obesity, and dental erosions. Their use should be limited to hydrating athletes after prolonged and vigorous exercise, and water should be the primary source of hydration for child and adolescent athletes.[83]

If your child participates in a sport, be proactive. If your team wants parents to provide snacks after games, talk to other coaches and families about instituting a fruit and water policy. Once Dr. Yum provided some ripe pears from the farmers' market after her son's soccer game. Her son, having seen the kids scarf down chips, cookies, and other processed treats after games, was worried about how the pears would go over with his teammates. Much to his surprise, they loved the pears and next season were asking him if his mom would bring those "awesome pears" again!

One other consideration when signing your young kids up for sports is how it will affect eating at home. So many families spend a lot of time in the car going to and from after-school activities like sports. With little time to get home and make dinner, they end up hitting the drive-through to get a fast meal for their hungry athletes. However, eating these low-nutrient meals may work against the benefits that the sports offer in the first place, and kids may be better off getting free play at home and a more nutritious meal. Here are a few solutions to avoid the drive-through on busy nights with sports and activities:

1. Feed kids early: Give them a big, nutritious meal or a super-sized healthy snack when they are hungriest, right after school. They are more likely to be able to make it home and have a lighter meal or snack after sports.

2. Plan ahead: Make a big meal the night before your busiest activity nights and save the leftovers. When you get home from sports, you can quickly have dinner on the table for your hungry athletes.

3. Pack healthy options: Take cut-up fruit and veggies with you for the ride home to tide kids over until you can get the rest of dinner on the table. Consider it the first course of dinner!

Making Your Children Aware of Food Advertising

In this era of intense, child-focused advertising, parents are not only having to say no to the latest toys and gadgets, but also to junk food. Food advertising is a monster business and the fast-food industry is a prime example. According to a report by the Yale Rudd Center for Food Policy and Obesity, in 2012, fast-food restaurants spent $4.6 billion in total on all advertising, a number that climbed significantly over the three previous years. Their report showed that the biggest fast-food advertiser spent $972 million, whereas the combined total of advertising dollars spent on all fruit, vegetables, bottled water, and milk was only $367 million. They also showed that kids from preschool to age eleven watched an average of three fast-food ads per day, while teens watched almost five fast-food ads per day.[84] Another study showed that for every hour of television watched, children see eleven advertisements for food, the vast majority being ads for high calorie, low-nutrient foods.[85] What these advertisers know is that branding works. Researchers found that when children were given five foods with fast-food labels and without, they preferred those with the labels.[86]

With advertising so prevalent, it seems logical that children's prolonged television viewing can adversely affect eating habits. One study showed that increased television viewing in teens was directly related to several unhealthy eating habits, including eating candy, eating fast food, and skipping breakfast, while the number of hours spent in front of the television was inversely related to fruit and vegetable intake.[87] Advertising also seems to affect subconscious eating. One study found that as children watched the commercial breaks during cartoons, they consumed 45 percent more snacks while watching food advertising than advertising for nonfood products.[88]

Having a television in the bedroom seems to compound the problem. The American Academy of Pediatrics recommends that kids watch no more than one to two hours of television per day (and no television before the age of two).[89] One study in New York found that 40 percent of one- to five-year-olds had a television in the bedroom, and that those kids watched more (4.6 hours on average) and were more likely to be overweight or obese.[90] This trend seems to continue into the teen years. A study of adolescents showed that those with a bedroom television reported more heavy television viewing (more than five hours per day), less physical activity, poorer dietary habits (including fewer servings of fruits and vegetables and higher intake of sugar-sweetened beverages), fewer family meals, and poorer school performance.[91] Advertisers are also getting more aggressive in marketing to kids, using toys, popular cartoon characters, interactive games, websites, and more. It's easier than ever for kids to fall prey to these pleas from food companies to buy their products.

What can parents do to counteract the pressure of advertising from food industry?

1. Talk to kids early about advertising. So many studies show that the effects of food advertising are seen as early as preschool. Talking to your preschooler early and often can help send the message that what we see on TV about food can be a trick to make us eat unhealthy food. Explain that the cartoon characters they see just help food companies be trickier and that the characters don't really eat the foods that they are promoting. Books like *Broc and Cara's Picnic Party* by Dave Wilson feature superheroes that show kids how eating healthy can be fun, and can counteract the advertising messages kids see on TV.

2. Limit screen time to less than two hours. Watch TV with kids when possible and talk about the programming and advertisements that you see. With advertising so pervasive on the Internet, it is also important to limit time on the computer, too.

3. Keep televisions and Internet access out of the bedroom. It's easier to monitor what programs your child is watching and how long he is watching when media viewing is supervised. When we see that kids have watched enough, then we can remind them it's time to get some physical activity.

4. Limit eating snacks or meals while watching television. Encourage children to be mindful eaters who pay attention to the sensations of eating. Food should be a social experience shared by family and friends where food is prepared and enjoyed together.

MAKING FOOD FUN FOR YOUNG CHILDREN

Food Passports for Food Explorers

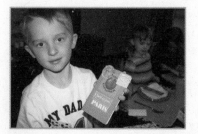

Parents can encourage kids to explore new foods by making a food passport with them. This can be easily done with a small notebook or journal and their picture. On DoctorYum.org, you can download a template that you can print and glue onto the front cover and inside cover. Add your child's picture, date of birth, and date of issue (the day you make the passport) to personalize it, and let kids decorate it how they like. Use a sticker or ink stamp to record when the child tries a new food, and write the name of the food and the country they "visited." Use the passport to record ethnic dishes that you try at restaurants, on vacation, or made at home. For younger or more reluctant eaters who may be still learning to eat simple foods, use it to record how they smelled, touched, or listened to a new vegetable as they chopped it. It's amazing to see how excited kids are to explore food if they get a stamp in their passport.

Salad Lab

For many kids, one of the last frontiers in food exploration is leafy green vegetables. By this age, many four-year-olds will happily eat carrots, corn, and green beans but may still turn up their noses at a salad or braised kale. One idea to help kids get comfortable with greens is to have a "Salad Lab." Kids love science and they love to create, so teach them a lesson in salad dressing that lets them concoct one that suits their own tastes. Give them a small mason jar and some ingredients to choose from. See the table with a simple formula for salad dressing. Once they add the ingredients, let them *shake* the jar! Kids will be much more willing to try fresh greens if they are topped with a dressing they made with ingredients and flavors they love.

SALAD DRESSING MAGIC FORMULA

HEALTHY FAT	+	SOUR	+	FLAVORS (or emulsifiers)
Olive oil Ripe avocado Avocado oil Grapeseed oil		Vinegars (apple cider, balsamic) Lemon juice Lime juice		Mustard Jam Honey Maple syrup Salt Pepper Herbs

Veggitos

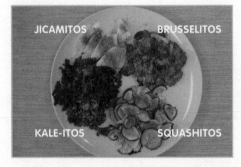

Kids love the taste of snack chips like Doritos. They are crunchy, salty, and savory with a blend of ingredients that keeps us coming back for more. Veggitos is a recipe that has been used in the Doctor Yum Project's kitchen to get tons of kids hooked on leafy greens and other veggies, and uses the same flavors found in our favorite snack chips.

The main ingredient in our seasoning is nutritional yeast, which is packed full of vitamins, minerals, and a cheesy, nutty flavor. Nutritional yeast is often found in health food stores and the health food sections of regular grocery stores (in bulk bins, most often). Sprinkle this blend on top of baked or raw vegetable chips and you have a winning flavor that will convert your most adamant veggie-hater. Once, at the Doctor Yum cooking camp, we sprinkled this seasoning on raw rutabaga slices and the kids were climbing on top of each other to get more! This works great with kale chips, Brussels sprouts chips, and raw jicama slices.

VEGGITOS SEASONING

¼ cup nutritional yeast

1 to 2 teaspoons sea salt (or pink Himalayan salt)

1 teaspoon chili powder

1 teaspoon cumin

1 teaspoon onion powder

1 teaspoon paprika

⅛ to ¼ teaspoon cayenne pepper (optional)

VEGGITOS INSTRUCTIONS

VEGGIE	PREP	BAKE TEMP	BAKE TIME
Squashitos	Thinly slice squash or zucchini (about 1/8 inch, a mandolin works great for this), place on a parchment-lined baking sheet and mist lightly. Sprinkle with seasoning and bake.	200°F	1½ hours or until crispy
Kale-itos	Rinse kale, remove thick rib and pat until very dry. Tear into bite-sized pieces. Massage all sides with very light cooking oil. Bake in a single layer until crispy and then season when finished.	350°F	About 7 to 10 minutes (some leaves may bake sooner, so check and remove the crispiest chips every few minutes so they don't burn)
Brusselitos	Cut off thick stem of several Brussels sprouts and let the outer leaves fall off until you reach the thick center (center can be saved for other recipes). Massage all sides with very light coating of olive oil. Bake in a single layer until crispy and then season when finished.	350°F	About 7 to 10 minutes (some leaves may bake sooner, so check and remove the crispiest chips every few minutes so they don't burn)
Jicamitos	Peel and thinly slice jicama into "chips." No baking necessary; just sprinkle with seasoning and enjoy!	None	None

MINDFULLY PARENTING THE SCHOOL-AGE CHILD

- Why your words are important
- Modeling behavior as a mindful parent
- Why movement has as much to do with brain function as burning calories
- Getting everyone on board

Choose Your Words Wisely: Drop "Picky" from Your Vocabulary

Many children in the preschool years still may not be eating all the foods their parents wished they would. It's not uncommon for us to hear a frustrated parent calling their preschooler a "picky eater." However, so many of these kids are still learning to eat new foods and need more exposure. Preschoolers are very aware of the language used around them, and hearing over and over that they are "picky" may lead them to live up to that label. Before calling your preschooler picky, consider that there are more positive ways to express that your preschooler is not yet eating a wide variety of foods. Try calling him an "exploring eater" or a "learning eater" to give him the idea that his food experience can grow and change with time. We train the teachers who use our Preschool Food Adventure curriculum to very carefully select the words they use to talk about food, so that kids understand that food preferences change and that learning to like new foods takes practice. The students are reminded that their taste buds need practice many, many times to learn to like a new food. The teachers also remind students to be nice when talking about food so that they don't hurt anyone's feelings. "Don't 'Yuck' someone else's 'Yum'" is how we explain it to the students. They are taught softer ways to talk about food they don't like, including "I don't care for that yet." When Dr. Yum visits some of the schools that are enrolled in Food Adventure, she often hears kids say, "I don't care for that. I have to keep practicing!"

Modeling Behavior

Showing our children how to live a culture of wellness outside of the home must involve modeling how we embrace a healthy lifestyle. If we impose one set of rules on our kids but then abide by a different set of rules, it can be confusing for children. They may be left thinking, "These rules must not be important if the grownups in my life don't follow them." Having food and drinks like soda in the house that adults regularly consume but are off-limits to kids will make them want them more. In a matter of time, they will find ways to get to those foods.

Modeling behavior doesn't mean that parents have to be perfect. So many of us struggle with maintaining healthy habits that perhaps were not established early, or life stressors have taken us off course. Show your human side, letting kids know that you sometimes have your own challenges with maintaining a healthy lifestyle. What kids will notice though is that you are trying. Your efforts will serve as a guide for living a healthy lifestyle.

One of our favorite tools for modeling healthy eating is the Rainbow Kit at todayiatearainbow.com. The kit includes a magnetic chart with rainbow and cloud magnets that represent different colors of food *the whole family* can try. That's the key to using charts—it's not about the reward; it's about the entire family getting involved in the journey to eat a rainbow every, single day.

Move! It's Good for Your Child's Brain

Lindsey Biel, MA, OTR/L, is an award-winning coauthor and a pediatric occupational therapist who shares her insight on why kids need to move in order to develop their brains as much as their bodies. As we first explored in chapter 2, "Young children first learn about the world through their senses." Biel explained it to Coach Mel this way:

They touch things, hear noises, experience smells and tastes, and explore their bodies' ability to move through space against the force of gravity. All of these pieces of sensory information blend together to give the child a secure understanding of the environment and their place in it. A solid sensory processing foundation empowers children to increasingly use their brains' thinking cortex for abstract, higher reasoning.

Today we ask very young children to sit still, look, and listen when their bodies developmentally need to *move*. Demands at school for "quiet bodies and active ears" bookended by hours of screen time—such as computers, smartphones, and game consoles—can contribute to childhood obesity, impaired cardiovascular health, decreased muscular strength and endurance, poor posture, headaches, neck aches, and vision issues. When kids are wired in to technology their relatively immobile nervous systems are not getting the three-dimensional brain and body stimulation that movement and sensory exploration provide.

Time and again, research shows that movement is essential to brain function. For example, having more than one recess period of at least fifteen minutes a day is associated with improved classroom behavior.[92]

Recess enables students to be less fidgety and more attentive to academic tasks, according to the National Association of Early Childhood Specialists.[93] Studies also show that physical fitness in school leads to better grades.[94]

How can you add more movement to your kids' daily life? Biel offers these suggestions:

- Have him sit on a physioball (which can be purchased from a sporting goods store or online) when doing homework or playing video games.
- Make sure she takes a stretch break every twenty to thirty minutes. You can use a kitchen timer, smartphone timer app, or if your child is on a computer, you can install the onscreen Time Timer software from timetimer.com.
- Take a flight or two of stairs instead of the elevator.
- Have her jump on a mini-trampoline while watching TV.
- Do "heavy work," using the big deep muscles of the body to push, pull, climb, crash, and jump. Incorporate this into everyday life: Have your child push the grocery cart

or a stroller full of toys, carry books, or play catch with a weighted medicine ball.

- Clean the house together, having your child spray non-toxic cleanser on surfaces and using large arm movements to wipe down. Let your child push the vacuum cleaner.
- Wheelbarrow walk from one spot to another, prompting your child to keep his back straight like a table. You may need to support him at his thighs or even hips to avoid having him arch his back.
- You don't have to be creative here to make movement fun. Get a card deck such as Move Your Body from superduperinc.com or play Twister, Cranium Hullabaloo, Simon Says, and so on.
- Be a good role model. Go biking, skating, swimming, skiing, horseback riding, or whatever you enjoy doing *together.*
- Dance!

You'll find lots more sensory smarts solutions for home and school in Biel's books, *Raising a Sensory Smart Child* and *Sensory Processing Challenges.*

Getting Everyone on Board

It can be difficult for children to establish healthy habits when family members are modeling very different priorities when it comes to wellness. This is especially true when children spend time in different homes, such as with grandparents who help with child care or with parents who are separated or divorced. It can be much harder for kids to learn the rules when they are inconsistent between households or between adults in the same household. When parents decide that wellness is important to their family, it's often helpful to verbalize that in a family discussion and make it official. A family mission statement can be a perfect way for you to take stock of what is important to your family and to have everyone in the family sign off on it.

Here is an example of a family mission statement: "The Wilson Family's Mission Statement: To create an inviting and supportive space for wellness. To provide opportunities for growth in leadership and education."

There are a number of values that you could include in a family mission statement, including wellness, education, giving back to the community, kindness, spirituality, or leadership. After listing those things that are important to you, let everyone in the family sign this statement, including your preschool-aged children. Display the statement somewhere prominent as a reminder for everyone to stay on track. You can download your own family mission statement template at DoctorYum.org or ParentingInTheKitchen.com.

 ### Coach Mel's Tip: Look Beyond Lunch

Parents tell me that lunch is typically the best meal of the day for picky eaters, even the older kids who aren't yet in full-day preschool or kindergarten. Typically that's because: (1) They skipped breakfast and are starving; (2) They get familiar and favorite foods most days for lunch; and/or (3) They eat best when in front of the TV or in the car between activities. "But at least they're eating," parents tell me. I understand, I do! However, if the goal is to help a child become a more adventurous eater, then the above tactics will backfire. Over time, try these three strategies instead:

1. Create a hunger schedule, not a hunger strike. (We talked about the importance of hunger in chapter 5.) In other words, parent consistently by offering predictable mealtimes with a variety of foods—three to four small samplings on a plate. "A little hunger is a good thing": It's worth repeating because it's crucial to success. This does not mean that if you let a kid get hungry, he'll eat anything. But if a child is *not* hungry, he is very unlikely to try a new food. *Too* hungry and kids gobble up only their favorite comfort foods, because they are too cranky to consider any other options. Starving is a bad time to try anything new.

2. Present at least one *new* food on his plate (with two to three small samplings of familiar favorites). If he protests, be calm and concise and say very matter-of-factly: "Yep, we've all got carrots on our plates today." Then, move on to a new topic. Say it once and don't revisit it, no matter how much he tries to object. Just learning to accept the presence of the food is the first step for many kids, even the older ones who may have hopped on the picky eater path. If the topic turns to learning about carrots and he informs you, "Hey, these are what Bugs Bunny eats!" then join in and come up with every fun fact you can think of:

- Did you know that the greens on carrot tops were once used to decorate the hats of royalty?

- Spiderman eats carrots so he can see better in the dark. He told me so.

- I can crunch this carrot louder than your father—listen . . . *crunch*!

3. Sit with your child, facing him, whenever possible and enjoy your meal together. Eating in front of the TV or staring out a car window with food from the drive-through is, at times, just a part of our lives. But the goal is to learn about new foods rather than be distracted from what we are eating. Ever sat in a dark movie theater with a huge tub of popcorn in your lap, and then at the end of the flick, been astonished that you ate it all? I doubt that if you had that tub in front of you while sitting at the table that you would have eaten the whole thing. Yes, a child will eat more volume when distracted, but she isn't progressing toward the long-term goal: an adventurous palate.[95]

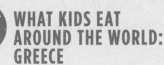

WHAT KIDS EAT AROUND THE WORLD: GREECE

In Greece, where one of the healthiest diets of fresh vegetables, olive oil, yogurt, and other traditional Mediterranean food has its roots, the culture is shifting. The influences of Western culture have settled in, and today Greece has one of the highest obesity rates in the world. The proportion of overweight children is now approximately 44 percent of the population.[96]

In a 2012 NPR interview, Jon Miller spoke with renowned New York University nutritionist Marion Nestle, who referred to the changing culture's "nutrition transition," blaming both human and economic factors on the phenomenon. "The nutrition transition happens very quickly," she said. "As soon as people get money, they start buying more meat and more processed foods. Well, that's fine if you don't eat too much of it. The problem is that we as humans, when we're confronted with large amounts of delicious food, we eat large amounts of food." Today, as Greece struggles financially, processed foods are now viewed as more economical. Miller reports, "With junk food so much cheaper than fresh food, they say, the lighter people's wallets, the heavier they'll get."[97] Still, where there's a will, there's a way, as Dr. Yum shares in the next story.

JIMMY'S STORY:
New Healthy Habits Lead to Big Changes

Dr. Yum once met an amazing young mother named Belinda at one of the shopping classes she taught. Belinda wanted to learn more about how to feed her seven-year-old son Jimmy better foods, but after hearing her story, it seemed amazing how far she and Jimmy had already come in their journey. Just a year earlier, his pediatrician labeled him "overweight," a diagnosis Belinda was not able to face when she first heard it. But when Jimmy had an unexpected health crisis directly related to his weight, she determined that their lifestyle had to change. She and her husband decided that they needed to make changes as a family and practice what they preach. So as they moved halfway across the country when Jimmy's dad got a new job, they also underwent a complete overhaul of their habits.

They stopped eating out and started to cook at home. They turned off the television and started sitting together at the dinner table. They incorporated more fruits and vegetables into their diet, and when Jimmy protested, they kept offering the same foods without wavering until his preferences changed. They were now living far from relatives who normally would indulge Jimmy with unhealthy treats, and they stopped letting him snack whenever he wanted and provided healthier snacks on a schedule. Each night they went on family walks until Jimmy felt strong enough to join the school running club.

The transformation was incredible, both physically and emotionally. At age six, Jimmy wore a size 10 to 12, but a year later he was wearing a size 7. He went from being self-conscious and introverted to gregarious and energetic. In school, he went from reading below grade level and struggling to keep up to being a top student. The family also reported that their change in lifestyle was great for their budget, too. By cooking at home and cutting out processed food, the family's food spending was cut by more than half! When asked the secret to their son's success, Belinda and her husband both said that in order for Jimmy to be healthy, the change had to start with them.

10

YOU CALL THIS A REST STOP?

Calming the Chaos of the School Cafeteria

Chances are it's been a while since you've ordered "hot lunch" in the school cafeteria. Whether you send a home-packed lunch with your child or they order lunch, eating in the cafeteria can be overwhelming at first. Coach Mel had a client who called it the "café-FEAR-ia" because the whole experience was a bit scary for him.

Imagine being a brand-new kindergartner, toting your sparkly new Disney Princess lunch box down the school hallway, when you turn and enter utter chaos. Older kids tower over you as you cross the sea of tables and try to find where you are supposed to sit for the next twenty minutes. Irritating fluorescent lights flicker while children chatter, teachers clap loudly to insist on silence, and rebellious kids ignore the adult plea and pop potato chip bags open with a *bang!* Metal lunch boxes clang as hungry tykes unpack a multitude of tins, cartons, juice boxes, and squeezable thingamajigs. The display on the tables is like a giant fire sale.[98]

Now picture the typical metal cafeteria table with benches made to fit the average fifth grader. Your kindergartner's feet are dangling and there's no backrest. She has to balance while her elbows hunch up practically to shoulder level in order to stabilize herself on the table edge, her little eyes barely able to see past the barrage of sandwich bags and containers spread before her. In an effort to ensure that their kids eat anything at all, well-meaning parents pack lunch boxes filled to the brim, typically with seven to eight different options.

She sits and tries to ignore the boy next to her who keeps elbowing her in the ribs as he turns to talk to his friend on the other side of her—and turns back to eat—and then turns back to his friend. By the time she gets out all the containers you've packed, plus the juice box straw finally unwrapped and poked hard enough that juice squirts her in the face, five minutes have gone by. She's holding up her other hand to signal the teacher, "Can you please open this lid?" but there are three other kids who need help first. Meanwhile, that nice girl that played with her at the craft table this morning wants to chat—and she just wants to make friends.[99]

Maybe she'll get a few containers open and swig down that juice, but now her mind is on recess. Here's the biggest dilemma: For most kids, their priority during that very quick lunch is to visit with their friends and get a few bites of food in in the process. However, teachers and the parents have a different priority for lunchtime: They want kids to have a nutritious meal so they are well fueled and ready to learn in the afternoon.

SOLUTIONS TO THE CHAOS

- Lunch-packing strategies
- Introducing new foods at lunchtime
- Find your way with a packing roadmap

If your school cafeteria resembles the picture we've painted above, and you want to rest assured that your child gets a healthy lunch in her belly, here are six solutions to finding some calm in the chaos:

1. Send one easy-open container plus a drink. Bento boxes are all the rage nowadays. For many families, there is just enough time to get lunches packed and to grab them on the way out the door in the morning. The solution is a one-piece bento with an easy-open lid. Bentos are not as overwhelming as a lunch box filled to the brim with individual plastic bags, containers, and drippy fruit cups with tricky foil lids.[100] Our favorites are EasyLunchboxes (the best-selling lunch-box system on Amazon) and the Yumbox (yumboxlunch.com). Both offer easy-open lids and compartments that are just the right size for kids. The Yumbox can be ordered with different trays that fit inside the box itself. Our favorite tray has five compartments each marked with a food group: Protein, Vegetables, Fruit, Dairy, and Grains to ensure a balanced lunch every time you pack.

2. Pack "grab and gab" food. Cut fresh fruit, veggies, sandwiches, cheese, etc., small enough so that kids can grab a piece without having to look down, and continue to gab with their friends across the table. Using a cookie cutter to create food in a fun shape like a dinosaur keeps the eating on track for some kids. But for kids that tend to eat a sandwich and skip the other items, try cutting the sandwich into small pieces so the child alternates grabbing a variety of foods, much like a mini-smorgasbord. Remember, you don't need to send a whole sandwich when sending half leaves room in little bellies for other key food groups.[101]

3. Include a power-packed smoothie that you made the night before. Freeze it directly in a cup or mason jar with a lid and be sure to include a wide straw. Wrap some rubber bands around the jar for added grip and to keep little hands from getting too chilly. By the time your child opens her lunch, the smoothie will be the perfect consistency, plus it helped to keep the lunch cold.[102]

4. Pack last night's dinner for lunch. If your child has a favorite healthy dinner, find ways to pack it in his lunch the next day. Use insulated containers to keep soups, stews, or pasta warm for lunchtime. Using leftovers can save time packing lunch in the morning, too.

5. Pack a waste-free lunch. A lunch-box system means that you won't be throwing away plastic bags every day. Use brightly colored cloth napkins and stainless steel water bottles to make lunch even more fun. Use lunch packing as a chance to show kids that they help to reduce, reuse, and recycle.

6. Start weekly lunch-box dinners at home. For kids transitioning to school lunch, introduce once-a-week "lunch-box dinners" where the entire family pretends to eat in the school cafeteria. At the entrance to the kitchen or dining area, one parent stashes a large bin, just like the kids will find at school. Each member of the family has their own distinct lunch box thrown into the bin, along with a few "old" random empty lunch boxes, so kids can practice digging down to the bottom to find their own. Once everyone is seated at the table, the child can practice the fine motor skills of unzipping zippers, unfastening Velcro flaps, and opening up containers. Choose a lunch box that is easy to open and pack it with "grab and gab" food, just like you would in the cafeteria. Once the meal is over, everyone latches their lunch box and puts it back in the bin, just like at school.[103]

Coach Mel's Tip: What's the Star of Your Child's Lunch?

As a speech-language pathologist, I teach the parents engaged in lunch-box dinners with their child to practice this little script: "I've got _____ in my lunch!" In all my years of sitting in school cafeterias and listening to young kids, it's always the first thing they say to each other. It's their traditional conversation starter, usually accompanied by them proudly holding up the celebrity food—the star of the lunch box. I can attest that I hear just as many kids enthusiastically say, "I have fruit today!" as "I have chips today!" Try for the veggies. It's really OK—it's just as cool to have vegetables cut up into stars or other fun shapes so they can announce, "I have *CUCUMBER STARS* today!" Better yet, get the kids involved packing the lunches and creating fun shapes so they can exclaim, "I made carrot triangles for lunch!" [104]

Dr. Yum's Tip: Avoid Prepackaged Lunches

Food companies have seemingly made things easy for us by creating premade lunches, with compartments filled with a complete meal including a dessert and drink. Your kids may ask for these because, of course, many of the packages are adorned with colorful graphics and familiar characters. Flip the package over and you may be shocked to find a laundry list of artificial preservatives and food dyes. One of the popular brands of packaged lunches also has as much as sixteen teaspoons of added sugar, which is almost three times what a young child should consume in a day.

Phasing in New Foods

When packing lunch, parents pray that their child will "just eat something!" But at the end of the day, especially if the child is a picky eater, parents sigh as they open the lunch-box latch and see that lunch has barely been touched. What can a parent do at home to encourage kids to eat lunch, even when they eat only five to fifteen different foods and are hesitant to try anything new? Here are some tips to encourage young eaters to explore beyond their preferred foods:[105]

1. Begin with exposure: Kids may need to see a new food multiple times before they may even consider trying it. That means they need to see it at school, too. If you're thinking, "But he won't eat it, so why pack it?" remember that the first step is helping your hesitant eater get used to the presence of that food in his lunch box again and again. Food doesn't have to be eaten to serve a purpose in food education, and it doesn't have to be a large quantity of food when first introduced.

2. Give kids ownership in the lunch-packing process. All kids like predictability and being a part of the process. Ask them to help with choosing, preparing, and packing lunch items. They are more likely to enjoy food when they are involved.

3. Include a favorite, but just enough: Most of us eat our favorite foods first, so be sure to include your child's preferred food, but not too much. Provide just enough so that you won't be worried that they are starving, but not so much that the other less-preferred choices don't stand a chance.

4. No comments, please! When the lunch box comes home, resist the urge to unpack it immediately. Give everyone a chance to breathe, especially those kids with sensory challenges who have difficulty with transitions from one environment to another. When you eventually open it, don't comment about the contents. Say nothing, positive or negative. For many kids, it creates too much focus on whether they ate or not. For now, just wash it out and set it on the counter for your child to pack again later that evening. If your child mentions the food or requests it again, that's the time to respond with a positive comment. Be careful not to say things like, "See, I knew you would like it!" You may mean well, but a child will typically interpret that as "See, I was right and you weren't." Try stating something positive, such as, "Pomegranates are one of my favorites—I like how they crunch and squirt at the same time in my mouth!"

5. Make a lunch-packing roadmap. Skip the filler foods like pretzels and chips and pack a balanced lunch by including items from all five food groups: proteins, grains, dairy, fruits, and vegetables. Use the chart below to keep you on track and have plenty of options that are frozen or shelf-stable in case you run out of fresh. See the packing map photo of a Yumbox container packed using our map. A handful of frozen edamame or dried fruit can be a great stand-in for fresh vegetables or fruit in a pinch. Whether you have a selective eater or a "foodie" with a palate that rivals a Top Chef, have all the kids in your family create a packing map and be responsible for their own lunch packing. Kids can choose foods from each group while the parent provides the healthy food options and keeps the kitchen stocked! Remember, it starts with exposure and builds from there.

LUNCH PACKING

Fruit	Grain
Mixed dried fruit	Whole grain bread
Raisins	Pasta
Grapes	Soba noodles
Berries	Quinoa
Apple slices	Pita bread
Melon balls	Torillas
Fruit and yogurt blend	Brown rice
All-fruit leather	Granola

Vegetable	Protein
Carrot sticks	Yogurt
Celery sticks	Lean meats
Edamame	Hummus
Sugar snap peas	Nut butters
Sliced sweet peppers	Sunflower butter
Cherry tomatoes	Beans, bean salads
Kale chips	Meatballs
Broccoli	Cheese
Vegetable soup	Eggs

Dr. Yum's Tip: Don't Forget Calcium

Kids need calcium for growing bones. Dairy foods like milk, cheese, and yogurt are a good source of calcium, but they are not the only way to keep bones healthy and strong. Nuts, beans, seeds, and leafy green veggies are also good sources of calcium that can also be packed into lunch. Hummus, which is made of chickpeas and tahini (sesame seed paste), is high in calcium and is a great lunch staple. Try a hummus wrap or cut veggies that your child can dip in hummus.

Coach Mel's Tip: Creating a Packing Map

To turn your hesitant eater into a lunch-box leader, create a poster board together that has a photo of the inside of her bento box, essentially creating a packing map that guides her to gradually adjust to new foods. Using colored markers, help your child list the foods she can eat with arrows pointing to where the foods go in the box. For example, the Yumbox lunch box has compartments with fun graphics representing dairy, grains, proteins, fruit, and veggies. Even if your child is limited to eating purees, write "applesauce" next to the fruit compartment on the poster. But also write a few more *future* purees that she needs to be exposed to, and put them in her lunch box occasionally, too. Parents and kids pack the lunch box *together* the night before, and the kids choose from their short lists what goes in each compartment. If they have exactly five preferred foods and there are five compartments, then we create a rule that they need to pick a new food for at least one of the compartments. Remember, this isn't only about eating, it's about introducing new foods through visual, olfactory (smell), and other senses. With just five nutritional categories, you can create endless combinations of grab and gab food.[106]

CASSIE'S STORY:
Finding More Focus in the Cafeteria

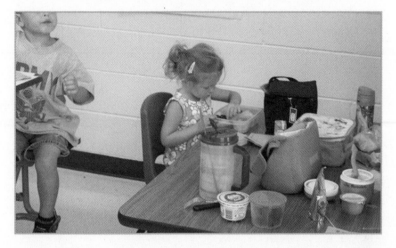

For a child who cannot adjust to the chaotic environment of the school cafeteria, Coach Mel has found that most schools are readily open to suggestions. For five-year-old Cassie, her school recognized the importance of lunchtime and how it impacts the rest of a child's day. Cassie was the tiniest child in the classroom and easily overwhelmed by noise, sights, and sound. Upon entering the cafeteria, the last thing she could do was focus on what her teacher needed her to do: eat.[107]

Cassie's principal allowed us to bring in a smaller table from the school library with chairs that not only fit Cassie, but most of her classmates, too. We positioned the table in the corner so that Cassie was flanked by a wall on her left and had two friends across the table. They also had a wall behind them to minimize distractions. Cassie's feet touched the ground, providing stability, and the table was at "sternum height" so her elbows easily rested by her food. Kids need core stability for fine motor skills like biting, chewing, and swallowing and opening lunch containers. "Right-sized" tables reduce noise, foster social skills at any age, and provide stability for the younger kids[108]

To make the experience even more efficient, Cassie brought her bento box. One easy lift-off lid and she is free to gab with her friends and grab bite-size pieces of fresh, yummy lunch. By the way, check out the pile of pandemonium on the rest of the table. How do those kids even find what they are supposed to be eating? No wonder half their food ends up back coming back home, uneaten. Oh, and see that bigger kid dangling his feet behind her? *That's* where Cassie used to sit.[109]

• •

Now that you have some tips on how to help your child deal with the chaos in the school cafeteria, we're ready to move on to navigating other outside influences like holiday meals and class celebrations.

11

NEGOTIATING YOUR PATH AROUND THE HOLIDAYS

From Halloween to Valentine's Day, the festivities and food treats can seem never-ending. Just when the last of the Halloween candy is consumed, Thanksgiving is upon us. After we venture through the December holiday celebrations, we get a brief reprieve thanks to New Year's resolutions, and then Valentine's Day parties stall our efforts to get back on the bandwagon once more. Sure, it's just a few holidays—over the course of four months. But if you have a child who is a hesitant eater or has food allergies or special dietary needs—or if you're just trying to stay consistent with a healthy lifestyle in your family—holidays bring a unique set of challenges. Sometimes family and friends may not understand the nuances of having a child who cannot eat what is traditionally served in their home. Sometimes family members go overboard indulging all of us in holiday treats. We'll help you negotiate your path and highlight some of the common issues that parents face at holiday celebrations and class parties, including birthdays.

HALLOWEEN

- Parenting Proactively: Strategies for keeping it fun and safe for all
- Parenting Mindfully: Keep expectations in check.

We love Halloween! It is a kid's nirvana—running from house to house with friends, holding on to plastic pumpkins, and shouting, *"TRICK OR TREAT!"* as neighbors offer an assortment of candies and toys to last for weeks. But what's a parent to do when their child with food allergies or special dietary needs so desperately wants to join in on the door-to-door fun? What ends up in their child's bag is vitally important for safety reasons. Here are a few strategies for parents to consider that may also be helpful if you're trying to reduce the sugar in your house:[110]

Strategy 1: Enlist the Help of a Few Neighbors

- Use secret passwords. Nobody wants a child to miss out on the big night. Most friends and neighbors will be thrilled to stash your candy alternatives by their front door. If your alternative treats need to be kept separate from other food substances, be sure to let them know. If your child is old enough and/or you're not present, just tell her that Mrs. Smith needs to hear the secret password (e.g., "monster mash") because she is saving something just for her. The last thing you want is Mrs. Smith accidently giving some random fairy princess your child's special allergen-free treat.
- Create a treasure hunt. Offer clues that lead your little pirate to the buried treasure where "X" marks the spot. Use brown grocery-bag paper and black ink and even singe the edges for that authentic treasure-map look. Give ten clues to ten neighbors; each piece of paper provides the next clue for where to go: "Yo ho ho, ye pirate gents! Go to the next house with the white picket fence!" Little does he suspect that the tenth clue will send him back to his own house, where he will discover a giant X and a special treasure buried beneath, just for him.
- Display a teal pumpkin. Food Allergy Research and Education (FARE) designed a unique campaign to raise awareness of food allergies by encouraging nonfood treats for

trick-or-treaters. Families can show support for the cause by painting a pumpkin teal and displaying it along with a printable sign from FARE to let children with allergies know there are nonfood treats available.

Strategy 2: Tangible Alternatives to Candy

Whether you're trying to avoid sugar or perhaps the top eight allergens, here are a few tangible alternatives to traditional candy.[111] You can plant a few of these with your kind neighbors or give them away to the little creatures knocking on your door that night:

- Eyeballs (and other spooky treats): Head to your favorite craft store to stock up on creative options for candy. A pillow sack of party favors, such as bloodshot Super Ball eyes, miniature magnifying glasses, Halloween stickers, or tiny decks of cards, is still a nice pile of loot for your little goblins to dump on the living room floor when they get home.
- Glow-in-the-dark bracelets: Activate all of them just before the doorbell starts to ring and put them in a clear plastic bowl so they give off an eerie glow when you open the front door. Trick or Treaters pop them on their wrists and run off to the next house, literally glowing. Besides, you can feel better knowing that everyone's kids are a bit more visible running around in the dark.
- Think outside the box: Most toy or craft stores have bins of whistles, harmonicas, and bubbles to replace candy. Don't forget small packets of origami paper, craft buttons, jewelry kits and beads, etc. There are aisles and aisles of wonderful candy substitutes that will keep your child busy long after the other kids' candy is eaten. Parents all over town will be eternally grateful to see something creative in their children's sacks rather than yet another pack of sour gummy worms.

Strategy 3: Get Rid of Excess Candy

Got too much candy? Here are two fun ways to get rid of it fast![112]

- Hold a candy auction: Dig into that Monopoly game and grab those pastel paper bills. Here's your child's chance to hold a candy auction! When all the bidding is over, he gets to count out how many paper bills (dollar amount is now a moot point) he received and trade those in for real money, but half goes into his savings account.
- Worth their weight in . . . dollars: Finally, a chance to use your bathroom scale and rejoice as the numbers go *up*! Kids get to weigh their loot and get paid $5 for every pound turned in. The next day, extend the family fun by going to the toy store or a favorite "haunt" to buy something together.

Coach Mel's Tip: Safety Considerations for Kids with Food Allergies

1. Separate candy. Make it clear to other adults if alternative treats need to be separate from other food substances due to cross-contact.

2. Bring an epinephrine injector. If you're not accompanying your child, make sure his friends know where the pen is stored and how to use it. If your child will be with friends in a different neighborhood than where you are, send two epinephrine injectors. On Halloween, it may take time for an ambulance to find your child and he may need more than one injection.

3. Allow trick-or-treating in a group only. As with all children, remind kids to stay together.

4. Give your child a fully charged cell phone with emergency numbers on top. Make sure her friends know how to use it, too.

Consider an app that can generate an image of emergency contact information and medical data for use as your child's phone lock screen. (Emergency responders can read this without unlocking your child's phone.)

5. Make sure your child is wearing an ID bracelet. It should be visible despite her costume.

6. Ask all children in the group to wait to eat their candy until it can be inspected at home. This is a general safety rule for all kids, but for those who have allergies, it also prevents accidental contact via another child during the excitement of trick-or-treating.

Expectations: Yours and Your Child's

Consider your own expectations and how those may in turn define your child's expectations for Halloween. Lori Lite, an author and national expert in childhood stress, assures parents, "It is not necessary for children to have the full-blown experience in order for them to have a good time"[113]

Ask your child what she would like to do. Perhaps she just wants to be in charge of passing out the glow bracelets while the two of you wear matching glow-in-the-dark vampire teeth! So often as parents, we try to do make a huge production out of a holiday because we feel we owe it to our kids. Funny thing is, most of the time, the kids are just thrilled to be a small part of it as long as they are sharing it with *you*.

So enjoy and be in the moment. Wear a funny hat. Tell a spooky story. Take lots of pictures and video, too. Stick a plastic spider on someone's chair at dinner. Don't be afraid to scream— it's the one night you can do so with abandon![114]

THANKSGIVING

- Establishing new traditions: Take the focus off the food.
- Parenting Bravely: The "what-ifs" that come from fear

You've reminded the relatives about your child's food allergies and done all you can to ensure that she is safe at the yearly family extravaganza. You've worked through the emotions that encompass the holidays, especially when dietary restrictions impact not only your little one, but your extended family as well. Time to focus on what Thanksgiving is truly about: gathering together with thankful hearts. It's about family, tradition, and community. It's about gratitude and giving. And yes, we express our thanks around the table, often with recipes passed down from generation to generation.

Take the Focus off the Food

How about establishing some new traditions for your child that don't focus on food, but on celebrating your time as a family, and ones that are centered on gratefulness and generosity? Here a few suggestions that put as much focus on family as the food:[115]

- Kids decorate the table: While the adults are preparing the food, let the kids have a special party to decorate the table. Older cousins can assist as the younger kiddos make the centerpiece, place cards, napkin rings, or place mats. This is a time to encourage each generation to get to know each other a little bit better. What wonderful conversation starters these will be when everyone sits down!
- A tisket, a tasket: Just before dinner, give everyone a small piece of paper. Each person writes down one funny fact about their lives, such as "My first job was at an ice cream shop and I'm lactose intolerant!" or "My husband called me by the wrong name our entire first date!" Put them in a small basket, perhaps decorated by your child, and while enjoying dinner, pass the basket around the table. Each person pulls out a piece of paper, reads it, and the table has to guess who wrote it. Then, that person tells the funny story in detail. This is the perfect game to record on camera—family history straight from the horse's mouth!

Make video copies and give them as holiday gifts in December. Family holiday shopping, done.

- Mr. Potato Head: Give the kids potatoes in various shapes and sizes, toothpicks, buttons, felt, and anything from the bottom of your craft box to create their own potato "turkeys," each with his own personality. Hint: Poke the potatoes with a fork in a few places, microwave them slightly the night before, and then refrigerate so that it's easier for little fingers to push toothpicks into the potato. These also make fun place cards.

- Play the Alphabet Thanksgiving Game: It's a lovely touch to share what you are thankful for, but here's a silly twist to do afterward. Go around the table clockwise and the first person must start with the letter A, then B, then C, etc. Always known for practical jokes, Uncle Rob might say: "I am thankful that Andy's pet snake hasn't escaped (yet) from the cage under the table." The child on his left might say, "I am thankful that Basketball season is coming, because I am going to score a gazillion points for my fourth-grade team!" or "I am thankful for Carrots because we dug up the last bunch at our Community Garden to give to the food bank."

When your expectations are out of sync with what your child may be capable of eating, it's natural to feel anxious at holiday celebrations. Focus on what your child *can* do and create memories together. A year from now, you won't remember how much turkey he ate—but you'll remember the smile on his face when he helped you set a beautiful table.

- Fresh herbs can decorate any platter or dish. Help your hesitant eater play an important role in creating the dish, even if she is not ready to taste it yet. She can decorate the platter with a variety of herbs, tearing the leaves to release the aroma and feeling the texture of the greenery in her hands. Remember to take a minute and admire the presentation.

"Ellie, I love the way you made a nest of greens for the turkey to rest upon. It makes the whole dish look beautiful!"

- Let children be the hosts. Letting the little ones arrange several small allergen-free vegetable trays, and then carry them from guest to guest as the adults help themselves, is a wonderful exercise in social skills. It creates the perfect opportunity for each adult in the family to chat with each child. So often, kids end up sitting together or playing in another room and miss out on the important feeling of belonging to the extended family.

Dealing with "What-Ifs" and Holiday Stress

Selective eater, hesitant eater, picky eater: These are all terms that describe children who fall on the spectrum of feeding challenges. Wherever a child falls on this spectrum, the holidays seem to raise the stress level for the child and her parents. When Thanksgiving and other food-centered holidays approach, the anticipation of an entire day focused on food has many parents agonizing over the possible outcomes when well-meaning relatives comment on their child's selective eating or a special diet. This time of year, Coach Mel tries to find practical ways to reduce the stress for these families. Some of the most common concerns from parents of kids with feeding challenges are as follows:[116]

- What if Junior won't take a bite of Aunt Betty's famous green bean casserole?

    It's not about the bite, it's about wanting Aunt Betty's approval. Focus on what Junior *can* do. If he can sprinkle the crispy onion straws on top of Betty's casserole, call Betty ahead of time and ask if he can have that honor. Explain how you would love for him to learn to eventually enjoy the tradition of the green bean casserole and his feeding therapist is planning on addressing that skill in time. But for now, she wants him to feel great about participating in the process of creating the green bean masterpiece. If Junior can't bear to touch the food because he has some tactile defensiveness, what can he do? Perhaps he can pick out the serving dish and escort Aunt Betty carrying the dish to the table? Taking the time to make Aunt Betty feel special by showing interest in her famous dish is all Betty and Junior need to feel connected.

- What if Grandpa Bob reprimands Junior for "wasting food" or not eating?

  Keep portions presented on the plate quite small—a tablespoon is fine. Many families use family-style serving platters or buffet style, where everyone dishes up their own plate. Practice this at home. It's not wasting food if Junior is practicing tolerating new foods on his plate. That food went to good use! If Grandpa Bob grew up during the Great Depression, this might be tough for him to understand. If he reprimands Junior, change the subject and tell Junior you're proud of him for dishing up one whole Brussels sprout! That requires some expert balancing and stupendous spoon skills!

- What if Junior gags, or worse, he vomits?

  Not surprisingly, this is the one sensory reaction that most relatives sympathize with and try desperately to avoid. Preparing the host ahead of time is gracious and appreciated. Coach Mel recommends that parents identify what stimuli are most noxious to the child and talk with the host about those, offering assistance in preparing special food or supporting the host's planned menu as much as possible. Bring a change of clothes for Junior, just in case, as well as a quiet activity for him to enjoy if you sense that the meal may be just too overwhelming for him. Plan other activities that don't involve food to emphasize the message of the season: being together, as a family.

DECEMBER HOLIDAY CELEBRATIONS

Whether you celebrate Christmas, Hanukkah, or Kwanzaa, winter holidays can be a lot of fun for families. They can also be a time when well-meaning relatives steer your family off course after you've already established healthy eating habits at home. There are ways to reinvent holiday traditions with a healthier twist. A favorite Christmas tradition is the Advent calendar, which counts down the twenty-five days until Christmas. Kids open a little paper door, one each day, to find a small chocolate. To encourage tasting and trying new healthy foods during the holiday season, the team at the Doctor Yum Project decided to put a healthy spin on the Advent calendar and make an "Advent-ure calendar" instead. Open each door to reveal a different fruit or vegetable each day. If there are hesitant eaters in your family, no worries! This can be fun for them, too. If your little ones are not ready to try each food by tasting, allow them to help you to prepare the food and build familiarity through other senses (taste, smell, etc.). This calendar can be downloaded in two sheets (cardstock recommended) from DoctorYum.org

Getting relatives on board with your culture of wellness can be delicate, especially during the holidays, when getting along with family is so important. But with some relatives, the sweet treats and unhealthy food shared with children can go overboard, and finding balance is essential. A proactive, soft touch is helpful when trying to combat a potential onslaught of junk food brought by relatives. Here are some ways to be polite yet proactive with your relatives at the holidays.

1. Brag good-naturedly about your kids. Tell your extended family how your kids have started to enjoy so many new and healthy foods and how they can't wait to show you the new recipes they are making at home.

2. Educate with love. Explain to family how so many kids experience diet-related illness; you're trying to make sure that your kids grow up with great eating habits so that they can have a long and healthy life.

3. Find ways to add healthy, flavorful dishes to your holiday table. Substitute a starchy side dish with a lighter vegetable side dish, like leafy greens, which are abundant in the fall. Try slow cooking collard greens with smoked turkey for added flavor. Pomegranate seeds are a fun autumn fruit that can be sprinkled over a winter salad with a brightly flavored pomegranate dressing.

4. Invite friends and family over to make new holiday "treats" that your kids enjoy. Let the kids be the star attraction so that the event and the kids are welcomed with open arms. Here's a great winter treat to make with relatives at the holidays: Sugar plums are naturally sweet with dried fruit, dates and honey, and a very fine dusting of superfine sugar makes them sparkle. Kids love using their hands to form them into little bites.

Sugar Plums

Makes about 36 sugar plums

¼ cup honey
2 teaspoons orange zest
1 teaspoon cinnamon
1 teaspoon allspice
½ teaspoon nutmeg (optional)
2 cups slivered almonds, toasted
¾ cup dried apricots, roughly chopped
¼ cup dried cherries
1 cup dates, roughly chopped
2 tablespoons superfine sugar

1. Mix the honey, orange zest, and spices in a small bowl.
2. Pulse the almonds in a food processor until they resemble a coarse meal. Add the dried fruits and dates and pulse several times, until chopped. Add the honey mixture and pulse until blended together.
3. Roll the mixture into dime-sized balls and roll each one lightly in sugar.

RETHINKING CLASS PARTIES

So many class parties can center on sweet treats and other unhealthy food. When you add up all the holidays and birthdays it may seem like eating unhealthy foods in school is more the norm than the exception. Here are some alternative ways to celebrate in the classroom that focus more on wellness and the celebration than sweets and treats.

Valentine's Day: Instead of focusing on chocolate and candy, why not make this a "heart healthy" day? Try sharing our Sweetheart Smoothie featured in chapter 8, page 177. While it's common for red sweets with artificial food dyes to carry the day, many kids are sensitive to these dyes and can have trouble concentrating after ingesting them. Instead, try using naturally red foods like strawberries, raspberries, and beets to color the day's foods. Let the kids enjoy a special class dance party to keep their hearts happy and strong.

St. Patrick's Day: A Green Dragon Smoothie (see page 177) can be renamed a Shamrock Smoothie that will leave the whole class feeling lucky. Swap out green cupcakes for green apples or green veggies served with spinach hummus. March is a great time to plant green veggie seeds in small pots. As a class project, kids can tend to these seedlings until the plants are big enough to transfer to a spring or summer garden.

Birthdays: Celebrate birthdays in class with some new healthy ideas like these:

- Let the child bring in a special song and have a ten-minute birthday dance party. The burst of activity will help them focus when they get back to their lessons.

- The child can bring in a favorite book for a birthday story time. She may enjoy telling the story of how the book became her favorite and feel special if her parent comes in to read it!
- Celebrate a child's journey around the sun. This is a Montessori tradition in which the child walks around a wooden sun placed on the ground to depict the years they have been alive. With each circle of the sun they share pictures or stories of themselves at each year of their life.
- If food is shared at class birthday parties, talk to the teacher about giving the parents some ideas for healthy party snacks. Fruit skewers, whole grain muffins, and vegetable and cheese trays are foods that will fuel kids steadily and healthfully so that they can get back to work after the celebration.
- In larger classes, the number of separate birthday celebrations may be overwhelming. One option is to let each child have a special privilege on their birthday, but combine celebrations for all the kids whose birthdays fall in a given month into one day.

Idaho mom Stacy Whitman decided to help her child's school develop healthy class parties and promote nutrition education in the classroom and the lunchroom. Her website, school-bites.com, chronicles the progress she has made in her community and is a great resource to find wellness ideas for schools, written materials like birthday agreements, and more. No matter what the celebration, it's most important to come together as a community or as a family and enjoy time together. Next, you'll find another mother's story on how she did just that.[117]

RAINA'S STORY:
In Her Mom's Own Words

Aimee is a mother to four-year-old Raina, her miracle girl who was born a micropreemie at twenty-four weeks' gestation. Aimee and her family embarked on an allergy-friendly journey after discovering Raina suffered from multiple food intolerances.

From the moment I step out of our car onto the snow-packed driveway of my aunt's house, my nose catches a whiff of the delicious aromas of roasted turkey, baked stuffing, and homemade pumpkin pies. The smell takes my mind and taste buds back, evoking all the warmth and nostalgia of Thanksgiving. But before my belly has a chance to rumble with the anticipation of gorging on the holiday spread, anxiety overtakes me. Will we be met with sly glances or unpleasant teasing again? Will my daughter's food intolerances consume the dinner table discussion? Will I be barraged from every direction with questions like, "I forget, what is gluten exactly?" and, "Now tell me again, why can't she eat this?" The knot in my stomach tightens. Am I prepared to handle the slew of well-meaning but clueless remarks, like, "Don't worry so much, a little won't hurt her"?

I am having second thoughts about being here. Maybe our family's dietary baggage is too great a burden to others. Should we even have come to this dinner? This might be as bad as when I took Raina to her friend's pizza party. I'm scared for her safety, afraid she may ingest the wrong foods. But it's not just the allergens, disguised in mouthwatering dishes and desserts, that I fear. My concern goes deeper: What if my daughter feels like an outcast, or that she feels somehow less of a person because she can't eat what others are indulging in?

My eyes turn to find Raina. She's skipping up the steps with glee. My Uncle Bob opens the door as full of high spirits as my little, bouncing girl. My aunts push him aside and run out with open arms and wide, glowing smiles to wel-come and hug Raina tightly. I relax for a minute; watching everyone's joy, my fears subside.

I remember the lessons that Melanie Potock, Raina's feeding therapist, taught us: Eating should be enjoyable and relaxed. It's as much about the act of sitting down and enjoying each other as the food. We aren't here just for the food. I take a deep breath, allowing myself a break from the overbearing stress I put on myself to manage these sorts of situations. As I let out a sigh, I remind myself of the pres-sure I place on myself to ensure Raina's safety and that I'm doing a great job.

As I waddle up the steps, laden with bags of my own allergen-free pumpkin pie, gluten-egg-dairy-free green chili cornbread, and homemade gravy, I think perhaps this year can be better. I inwardly repeat my daily mantra, "It's getting easier each day. It's getting easier each day."

Aunt Margie jolts toward me to grab a bag and, peeking in, says, "Oooh, look as these goodies! Your cousin Lizzie will be so happy. She's on some crazy diet, off the dairy and gluten as well."

"Really?" I reply in shock. I burst into a big smile, eager to greet my cousin, our new comrade on our allergen-free team.

While I may not always have faith that my family or friends will understand Raina's needs or bend over back-wards to accommodate her, I can hope that each year will improve as we all grow. I'm certain Raina will someday grow to be her own advocate and we, as a family, will find improved ways to cope with our stresses. Now, that is something to be thankful for!

(12)

THAT'S NOT WHERE I WANTED TO GO!
Food Allergies and Other Medical Conditions

∙∙∙

We cannot write a book on parenting and feeding without sharing some of the unexpected detours that many parents face when their child has feeding challenges. There are a multitude of reasons that families struggle with food and one of the most common is when a child must be on a special diet because of food allergies, intolerances, or medical issues. Examples include celiac disease, food protein-induced enterocolitis syndrome (FPIES), and feeding difficulties related to sensory processing disorder, as well the conditions of eosinophilic esophagitis, life-threatening food allergies, and type 1 diabetes, which are described in this chapter. The name of the disease or disorder is not as important as the common denominator for all of these families: The stress associated around feeding their child is palpable. Each family we interviewed reported that educating other parents was key to building a community that is sensitive to every family's challenges. We hope that the stories in this chapter raise awareness and encourage more families to support one another, because each child's journey is influenced by community support and understanding.

EOSINOPHILIC ESOPHAGITIS

According to the Mayo Clinic, eosinophilic esophagitis (e-o-sin-o-FILL-ik uh-sof-uh-JIE-tis), or EoE, occurs when eosinophils (a type of white blood cell) builds up in the lining of the esophagus, inflaming and injuring the tissue. A chronic immune system disease whose incidence has increased significantly over the past two decades, eosinophilic esophagitis is now considered a major cause of digestive system illness. Symptoms in children include difficulty feeding or swallowing, vomiting, abdominal pain, no response to "reflux" medications, and malnutrition and poor growth.[118]

Erin is the mother of Gavin, now in middle school. When Gavin was fourteen months old, he was diagnosed with failure to thrive, a label that reflected how his growth had stalled but did not provide answers why. In his first year of life, Erin says, Gavin "was screaming all the time—truly all the time"—and sleeping in ninety-minute stints. Erin was up with him around the clock, trying to determine why he was in so much pain. Further complications ensued as Gavin began to eat more solid foods and began having caustic bowel movements that resulted in severe blistering on the buttocks. Medical tests ruled out disease after disease, until finally, at twenty-two months of age, he had completely stopped growing. Erin describes it this way: "His hair, his fingernails, his whole body—*everything*—everything stopped growing."

Shortly after age two, Gavin was finally diagnosed with eosinophilic esophagitis. A gastroesophageal disease exacerbated by both environmental and food allergens, EoE is an emerging health care issue that has increased two- to tenfold over the past ten years. In fact, the American Partnership for Eosinophilic Disorders estimates that the prevalence is greater than one in 2,000 individuals.[119]

Little Gavin was treated with six months of inhaled steroids, reflux medications, and more. Eventually, when he was three, he had a special surgery called a fundoplication, which prevented stomach acid from rising up into his throat (esophagus). Because he was able to drink a specialized formula and eventually begin to eat a few solid foods while gradually gaining weight, he avoided a gastrointestinal tube to deliver nutrients directly to his stomach. However, many children with EoE need these tube feedings to grow and thrive.

Erin explained how her emotions around the disease developed over time: "When I look back at that time period, there were so many things going on as a parent. Everything in the community centers on food—birthdays, family get-togethers, and play dates over lunch with the kids. When you're in that environment and your kid can't eat anything and doesn't have the energy to play, well, the social piece was very difficult. There were so many times I would just cry afterward and I was so tired! It was exhausting having to explain the disease every single time I met someone new. I just wanted him to be like the other kids—I wanted to be like the other parents."

Coupled with those feelings was an underlying emotion: fear. "I had a lot of fear and I didn't want to project that onto Gavin. I had to monitor each day's events because just one tiny accidental taste would put him back on steroids and medication. I did not want to go back there, but we often did." Plus, life had its own unique complications, especially when traveling. Erin didn't know if certain foods would be available when traveling, so she always brought an extra suitcase packed with foods Gavin could tolerate, plus medications. "Going through airport security was always a big deal—there was so much explaining and documentation necessary." Bringing specific foods into restaurants created problems, too. "There were several times when we were asked to leave a restaurant—even though my husband and I were paying customers—because we had brought in our own food for Gavin."

And then there was school. Erin was very concerned about how she came across to other parents, especially those that didn't understand the gravity of the disease. Gavin's symptoms were easily triggered by not only food, but also by what chemical was in the modeling clay in art class or what cleaning product the janitorial staff used to wipe down the desks and floors. He would often come home with blisters around his mouth and enlarged lymph nodes from the tiniest exposure. "It took time to educate teachers, school staff, and other parents just how severe EoE can be and truly get them to understand. It's a hard road and I was worried that I appeared demanding. But I'd bring in pictures of the blisters or even an inflamed esophagus—a picture is worth a thousand words—and they would get it."

Comparing the healthy versus unhealthy photos made it more real for the other adults—but the comparisons to other kids were a painful reality for Erin and her family. "Year-round, I'd watch the other kids his age at the park and see them able to jump, run, swing, eat their entire meal in one sitting." Erin longed for that, especially for Gavin. "I'd see chubby little legs and faces and hands and dread having people ask, 'Why is your kid so small and skinny?' I'd get in my car and cry." Eventually, Erin began to see that they were making progress and that Gavin was beginning to thrive. "Just getting the right diagnosis and then the right balance of the various medications—that made a big difference for us. And the fear—it's always there, but each year we peel back the layers of emotions. Each year there is more hope because new medical breakthroughs are happening," and more people are aware of how to help.

After years of so little sleep and constant worry, Erin can now look back and tell other parents what helped her the most: having one individual outside the family who could provide respite care. "Just one person other than your spouse who can walk that walk with you. If you don't have that, the worry will consume you. You'll lose yourself and you'll lose your relationships with the people you love. I'm very grateful for my friends who supported me through the tough times." It's about community.

LIFE-THREATENING FOOD ALLERGIES

One in thirteen children have a life-threatening food allergy—or allergies. According to Food Allergy Research and Education, "a food allergy results when the immune system mistakenly targets a harmless food protein—an allergen—as a threat and attacks it."[120]

Keeley is mom to "Little Miss," who was diagnosed with a serious peanut allergy as a toddler. Their unexpected journey began when Little Miss was about one year old and she was first exposed to peanuts in her day care, where the children were engaged in a peanut butter craft. Fortunately, she didn't ingest the allergen, but after just touching the peanut butter, she immediately broke out in hives and swelling. Allergy testing revealed that Keeley's daughter could not ingest peanuts, tree nuts, dairy, or gluten. To add to the situation, Little Miss also had significant challenges adjusting to a variety of food textures and became a selective eater. She would only eat three different foods, was allergic to many others, and life began to get very, very complicated.

In addition to receiving occupational therapy and speech therapy to address these feeding challenges, Keeley took matters into her own hands and decided to focus on parenting proactively. She began to network, meeting other parents of kids with food allergies in her community and online. Keeley reports, "That's how I first learned about cross-contamination: Other parents taught me that foods that I thought were OK for my child to begin to try, actually were not." Hidden allergens can be dangerous and manufacturers are not required to notify consumers if their product is manufactured on the same machinery or in the same facility as potential allergens. Statements such as "manufactured in a plant that also manufactures peanuts" are strictly voluntary. Just because a parent doesn't see that statement on the packaging doesn't mean there is not a risk of cross-contamination.

Keeley practiced compassionate parenting, using a respectful and caring approach as she helped guide Little Miss. For most food allergy parents, day-to-day precautions become the norm. "You forget that something's different about your child. But then I'd have those moments when a party or community outing was not a safe environment for her and I couldn't allow her to attend." Keeley describes her emotions: "My heart would break for Little Miss, because as a parent I knew she was missing out. This past summer she went to Camp Blue Spruce, which is a food allergy camp for kids. She went overnight, and she was safe! She got to have those camp experiences that I thought she would never be able to have. It was overwhelming for me—I cried a lot—out of happiness for her."

Sometimes, it was clear to Little Miss that she was not invited to friends' birthday parties because other parents were frightened of the possibility of Little Miss having an allergic reaction while under their care. Keeley did her best to invite other parents and their kids over to her home first. "I wanted to show them it's OK. I'd explain that I'll send her to their house with safe food, and although they still needed to keep an eye on the situation, they would appreciate that I was not trying to make them figure it all out. I tried to do it in a positive way and build relationships with other parents in our community so that I [didn't] come off as demanding. Consequently, I feel like I have partners in this process."

Still, the fear is always there, especially in a new and uncertain environment. Now that Little Miss is getting older (she's in elementary school), it's easier because she can advocate for herself. Keeley explains, "If I see her fearful, which is unusual because she's typically very calm about it, that's when it's the hardest. One day she asked, 'Why did God give me food allergies?' When she's having a challenging time with it—that's when I'm hurting for her." To parent bravely, Keeley takes a deep breath and tries to be calm in order to keep Little Miss calm. She finds strength in support groups where she can vent about the trials of the day, get constructive feedback, or hear ideas for approaching a challenging situation.

Keeley, who blogs about her experiences at keeleymcguire.com, suggests these three tips for parents who are new to this journey:

1. Always be sure your child carries *two* epinephrine injectors, because you may need the second one before an ambulance gets to your child.
2. Research, research, research! Know exactly what is in your food.
3. Use snacksafely.com for the most current list of snacks that are free of peanuts, tree nuts, and eggs.

TYPE 1 DIABETES

Type 1 diabetes in children (once termed juvenile diabetes) is a medical condition where a child's pancreas no longer produces the insulin needed to survive. Complications from the disease can develop over time unless blood sugar is managed on a daily basis. According to jdrf.org, "Each year, more than 15,000 children and 15,000 adults—approximately 80 people per day—are diagnosed with T1D in the U.S.[121]

Julie Kay, a mother of four, has three sons who have type 1 diabetes, all diagnosed when they were toddlers or younger. In fact, her youngest boy, Gabriel, was diagnosed at just eleven months of age.

Julie Kay reflected on the heartbreak of getting the diagnosis for her oldest son when he was two years old. Jonathan's symptoms of excessive thirst and frequent urination were an immediate red flag to her husband, a pediatrician. What followed for Julie Kay was a crash course in type 1 diabetes—and learning that her child was at risk for developing serious complications, including kidney, eye, and nerve damage. She jumped in with both feet and learned how to manage the disease for a two-year-old until he could, one day, implement those same strategies on his own. At that time, it was believed that any children they might have in the future would only have a 5 percent chance of having diabetes.

Then, Benjamin was born. Parenting proactively, his parents decided to include their infant in a research study that was designed to determine if a child who had a sibling with type 1 diabetes would indeed develop the disease. Soon, the study revealed that the diagnosis was inevitable, and with some experimental intervention, the onset of Benjamin's disease was delayed until just after the age of two. Meanwhile, little Gabe was born and received the diagnosis before age one.

Julie Kay now found herself seated around the dinner table with her oldest child (a daughter) and three boys ages eight, two, and one, all in different stages of feeding development and with type 1 diabetes. She remembers that each child's sensory system was unique and all three boys experienced their own stages of picky

THAT'S NOT WHERE I WANTED TO GO!

eating, mostly related to texture. This made the situation even more complicated and stressful. She recalls, "I remember days when I would be standing at the pantry and thinking, 'What am I going to feed these kids?' and there would be tears in my eyes."

Julie Kay personified parenting bravely and resolved never to let her kids see her sweat. "I was determined that I would raise them in such a way that they would not hate their disease," and that included keeping mealtimes as relaxed and happy as possible. "The more negative things that happened to them due to this disease, the more they might rebel against their disease when they got older." Julie Kay took on full responsibility for managing their symptoms until the boys could begin to learn to do finger pricks and shots on their own. Instead of calling them into the kitchen for one of the many finger sticks to draw blood and test glucose levels, Julie Kay quietly joined them where they were. "If they were in the living room building Legos," she says, "I would quietly approach them with whatever the need was"—a juice, a finger prick, a shot. She maintained control of the disease rather than having the disease control her family.

But when it came to eating, the boys *had* to eat. Initially, the boys did not have insulin pumps to automatically regulate their insulin levels and they needed frequent meals focused on carbohydrates and protein. Julie Kay knew exactly how many carbohydrates were in the boys' favorite foods like the back of her hand. The stress was often overwhelming, but the fear was worse, particularly when the boys went to friends' homes or special school events.

Class parties were the hardest. There were days when Julie Kay was tempted to keep her eldest son home from school because there was just no controlling the mountains of sugar that other parents brought into the classroom for parties or holiday functions. He often had to eat something different than the other kids, and no one wants their child to be singled out in a group like that. Over time, as the school began to incorporate healthier options into classroom celebrations, life got easier. Once the boys had insulin pumps, even birthday parties were more manageable. Still, Julie Kay had to call the hostess, often whom she had never met, and explain her son's feeding challenges. When her boys arrived for the party, they not only had a gift for their friend, they had a laminated card for the birthday child's parent with emergency information in case of an unexpected change in blood sugar.

Play dates and outings could also present the unexpected. An emotional turning point for Julie Kay was the day that Jonathan was invited to go sledding up in the mountains with a friend's family. The plan the family shared with Julie Kay was that they would have lunch followed by sledding. But at the last minute, they reversed the order and went sledding first. The lunch afterward was not enough fuel to balance the day's exercise, and Jonathan had a seizure (due to low blood sugar) on the car ride back down the mountain. If he had just had a snack while riding in the car, Julie Kay would not have received the phone call that every parent dreads: "We have your son in an ambulance." It was one of the most frightening experiences in her life.

How did Julie Kay learn to let go of the fear over time? She didn't. It's impossible to let go entirely because the disease is always there and the outside world is unpredictable. "Preparation . . . and I relied on my faith a lot," she says.

Food is the center of most community events and the focus of time together as a family. Every day, Julie Kay checked in with herself and asked, "How are we going to get through this day and make it the best possible day it can be?" One way to do that was to never argue over food. That was her golden rule. "I wanted my kids to be happy and as healthy as any other kid," and to do that, she parented compassionately. Now that the boys are older, they have learned to have the same compassion and make sure to call her on a daily basis while away at college. "That's unusual for boys!" she laughs. "It's typically a quick check-in call just because it helps me to hear their voice," and then, she turns their day and their disease over to them. Over time, they have all learned to manage diabetes. During a recent photo shoot for a campus project, Ben was asked to write one word somewhere on his body that personified his life. He chose "persevere" and scrolled it across his abdomen. The word was flanked by his glucose monitor on one side and his insulin pump on the other.

WHEN A CHILD
NEEDS MORE HELP
The Role of a Feeding Therapist

Sometimes, our path in life includes a few detours. If these feeding strategies aren't working as well as you hoped, your child may benefit from a feeding therapist to get back on the road to adventurous eating. Whether your child has special needs or is a kid who just can't seem to climb out of a picky eating rut, seeking help can ease the stress that your family is feeling at mealtimes.

Feeding therapy covers a wide range of abilities and addresses the physiological, sensory, motor, and behavioral skills necessary for progressing through the developmental process of eating. Feeding therapy is never just about the child, because the act of feeding is a reciprocal experience. It's about the entire family and establishing what many of us take for granted: enjoying mealtimes, restaurants, cooking, and food experiences together, with joy, on a daily basis. Let's face it: Food is love. Life revolves around sharing food together. When a child is not able to enjoy a variety of foods at mealtimes, it impacts the entire family. It changes social situations with friends. It influences the child's behavior at school and in society. It's not a road anyone wants to go down, but sometimes, it's unavoidable.

"I never imagined my child would have trouble eating." Those words are often the first comments that parents have for Coach

Mel when they ask about feeding therapy. Most parents don't realize that 25 percent of the general pediatric population presents with feeding difficulties.[122] With the survival rate of premature infants increasing in at least the past twenty years, the need for specialized support around feeding challenges inherent to preemies has also increased. With one in sixty-eight children diagnosed with autism spectrum disorder (ASD) in 2010,[123] the need for feeding therapy for children with ASD has increased significantly since the 1990s. Regardless of a child's diagnosis or lack of one, we understand that for any child living in a chicken nugget world, learning to be an adventurous eater isn't always an easy journey.

SYMPTOMS THAT INDICATE FEEDING THERAPY MAY BE HELPFUL

Feeding therapy can be beneficial for children of any age. There are many reasons for seeking support, and here are some of the most common.

Infants[124]

- Feeding your baby is not an enjoyable experience. It's difficult and stressful. A feeding therapist is a feeding detective and can help you figure out why.
- Baby is not gaining weight. A feeding therapist will collaborate with your pediatrician and other professionals, such as a gastroenterologist, to examine all the possible factors. Sometimes, when a baby is not consuming enough calories, it is due to physiologic, oral motor, or sensory issues that prevent baby from sucking effectively on the breast or bottle. The feeding therapist may also collaborate with a certified lactation consultant or have those credentials, too.
- Baby is having trouble transitioning to purees or solid foods. Learning to suck purees off a spoon or fingers is part of the developmental learning process and eventually

leads to more advanced skills, like chewing. There are many reasons that babies stall here and catching it early is essential. If your baby is not adjusting to age-appropriate solid foods by eight months of age, talk with your pediatrician and consider feeding therapy.

- Baby gags and/or vomits on a daily basis. The occasional gag is nature's way of protecting baby's airway until she can control the pieces of food in the mouth. However, daily gags can lead to daily vomiting and discomfort, which leads to baby learning that eating is not fun. A feeding therapist can determine why your baby is having trouble and offer strategies to help overcome a sensitive gag reflex.

- Baby has not begun to drink from an open cup and cup with a straw by one year. By this age, babies should be developing a mature swallow pattern. Babies drink (and swallow) from the breast or bottle differently from the way older children drink from an open cup or straw. Having an experienced feeding therapist to offer advice can make all the difference.

Toddlers[125]

- Feeding your toddler is frustrating. "He won't sit in his high chair." "He spits out his food and just wants milk." "He throws his plate, his food, his cup—I dread feeding him!" There are many reasons that kids behave the way they do, but a speech-language pathologist, occupational therapist, or a feeding-trained board-certified behavior analyst (BCBA) who specializes in feeding skills can help you determine *why* your child is behaving this way and what to do about it.

- Your toddler hasn't grown much. Your child hasn't yet been diagnosed with "failure to thrive," but your instincts tell you it's time to seek help. Failure to thrive is a specific medical diagnosis with criteria on how much a child's growth has stalled. But many pediatricians wisely refer kids who are not taking in adequate calories to feeding therapy even before the criteria has been met.

- Your toddler seems especially picky. A feeding evaluation will tell you two things—first, if it's typical, age-appropriate picky eating, and second, how to prevent this particular stage in toddler life from becoming a problem in the near future.

- Your toddler eats great at school, but not at home. That's great! It means she is capable! Feeding therapy, especially when the evaluation and treatment are conducted in the home, can pinpoint why a toddler is a more hesitant eater in the home than in other environments. Another example is the child who cannot tolerate eating in restaurants. Many times, the restaurant is too stimulating for their sensory systems. Therapists trained in sensory integration can give specific strategies that will open the door to new dining experiences.

- Your toddler refuses to eat anything but his favorites. "He likes chicken nuggets, macaroni and cheese, and French fries, so that's what I give him." This is a common dilemma parents and therapists encounter when a child is age three. Toddlers often go on "food jags" where they insist on eating the same foods, over and over. Problem is, they eventually get tired of eating the same thing and the list of preferred foods dwindles. A feeding therapist can offer suggestions on how to broaden the variety of foods that he is willing to try, and eventually, learn to enjoy.

Preschoolers and School-Age Children[126]

- His siblings label him "the picky eater of the family." Kids will most often live up to labels we assign to them: "Oh, he's our math whiz," or "She's our little athlete," or "He's our picky eater." A feeding therapist can help "your picky eater" begin to think of himself differently and have the confidence to try new foods.

- Your child has food allergies. One of the challenges that parents encounter when their child has food allergies is what to offer and how to expand a child's food preferences while keeping them safe. Be sure the therapist you choose has extensive experience with children with food allergies and food intolerances.
- Your kid won't eat in the school cafeteria. Ever been to a crowded school cafeteria? It can be overwhelming in so many ways. Feeding therapists are often welcomed into schools to provide strategies for both the child and the staff, so kids can eat a relaxed lunch with their friends and get some important nutrition before academics start that afternoon.
- Your child wants to eat the same food as his friends but never learned to like that food. This is more common that you might expect. Coach Mel had a teenage client who wanted to get a hamburger or pizza with his buddies after football, but he had grown up in a vegan household and hadn't been exposed to that type of food. Plus, due to sensory issues as a child, he had a very limited repertoire of food he could tolerate without gagging. His parents were very supportive and wanted him to make his own decisions about a vegan lifestyle. He may decide to adopt the vegan lifestyle again someday, but being able to eat with his friends was very important to him at this age. Likewise, older kids who only eat chicken nuggets or macaroni and cheese limit themselves when the other students at school are hanging out at restaurants and food-centered events.

Whatever the reason, whatever the age, there is support for your child and your family and stress-free mealtimes are possible. If you just have *one* meal per day together, in the course of childhood that equates to over six thousand meals you'll be sharing. If you need an extra guide on this journey, a feeding therapist is one of the professionals who can help. Take it one step at a time.

DAVID'S STORY:
In His Mom's Own Words

When my son, David, was three years old, he reduced his edible repertoire to two items: French fries and potato chips. At first, as he refused more and more foods, I assumed he was just a "picky eater," like all of my friends' kids were around that age. But before long, his percentiles for weight were sinking faster than the Titanic, and his hair had become the consistency of steel wool. He also refused to eat in front of peers, or in any situation that was new or otherwise uncomfortable for him. So by the time we got down to the short list of refined potato products, I was in anguish, powerless, and walking on eggshells all the time. I read books; I consulted nutritionists and cooks; I tried anything and everything I could possibly think of to get some food down.

Looking back, I am amazed at what developed. Each feeding was a varied combination of presenting the food, waiting, watching, begging, pleading, cajoling, ignoring, bargaining, threatening, waiting some more, and then finally giving up. Meal after meal, we both ended up tired, frustrated, and generally upset. Our mealtime could be up to one and a half hours long—and there were three or more sessions per day! So many opportunities for failure! It was not long before I surrendered to hopelessness and to the certainty that there had never been a parent so lacking in skill and maternal instinct.

This was the state of affairs when Melanie, our feeding therapist, arrived at our table. After just a few minutes of observation during dinner, Melanie took me aside and offered what I later understood to be her most important words of advice. She told me to relax, to show my son that everything was OK, and to be open to the possibility that eating can be fun. She then instructed me to replace my "worried mommy" face with a "happy" face of eager anticipation. This was not an easy feat, as I was sure we were on an irreversible path to death by starvation. Yet she assured me that three meals of French fries per day was still a long way from a feeding tube, and a feeding tube was still a long way from death, and so I gradually I began to breathe again. Per Melanie's instructions, I pasted on the "happy" face and luckily was pretty convincing. And when I saw how my sense of ease in turn relaxed my son, I understood that change for him began with me.

For us, the process was very slow. It took weeks for my son merely to tolerate having a new food sitting on the same plate as the French fries. Then we worked on getting him to touch it, to hold it to his lips, taste it, eat it, and finally to eat it without a major fuss. Expanding his menu required hundreds of tiny steps, a time-consuming process to be sure, but one that created many opportunities to celebrate success along the way. In fact, despite his phobias, mealtimes gradually became fun times—for all of us. My son's favorite food game was to see what ridiculous thing he could get us to do by trying a new food. Daddy's barefoot ballet in the snow was a sure bet for a big bite!

My son now eats his "three meals a day plus snacks." He is not a perfect eater, but he'll eat from all the food groups, he has regained his percentiles in weight and height, and now will eat at school, in restaurants, and even at birthday parties. When he occasionally objects to a food, the hairs still habitually raise up on the back of my neck. But now I have learned to put on a grin, join him in lamenting the horror that his life has become, and confirm that he is surely the unluckiest child in the world to have a parent that would serve him this completely inedible mound of so-called food. Then we laugh and move on to another subject while enjoying each other's company over dinner.

I must also add that with my second child, now six years old, eating was a completely different story, thanks in large part to the tips that Melanie shared. My daughter began eating by feeding herself, making a mess, and delighting in the mealtime process. She still meets new foods with enthusiasm and eats heartily and healthily. Just last night she declared, "Mom, the asparagus is really extra delicious tonight!"

Having experienced firsthand the trauma and drama of a child who will not eat, I want to reassure parents that whether your child's challenges are physical or psychological in nature, whether your child is a picky eater or you just want to develop healthy attitudes toward eating, it can be done—step-by-step. Children can learn to eat well, and we can all learn to have fun eating together![127]—*David's mom*

. . . .

FEEDING THERAPY: FREQUENTLY ASKED QUESTIONS

Whenever children stall in their feeding progress for more than six weeks or when it is impacting nutritional status and/or growth, a feeding assessment is warranted. Let's address some of the most common questions that parents have when considering feeding treatment.

1. Who seeks out feeding therapy?[128]

- Owen, an adorable baby who was breast-fed at home but having difficulty with bottle-feeding at his day care, was irritable and losing weight. His mother felt guilty for not being with him and the day care worker tried to support her by saying, "When he's hungry enough, he'll eat!" But no one had realized he had a posterior or submucosal tongue-tie, which is not always easy to detect. He was hungry and wanted to drink from the bottle, but he wasn't capable.

- One-year-old James was gagging on any food that wasn't a smooth puree. The repeated gagging was making mealtimes uncomfortable for him and sometimes the gags would cause him to vomit. His mother had been feeding him away from the rest of the family, so as not to "gross out" her husband and kids. They rarely had family dinners together.

- Isaac's parents were at their wits' end. Isaac, age four, who had autism and sensory processing challenges, had reduced his repertoire of acceptable foods to five things: potatoes, French fries (but only a specific brand), chips, milk, and juice boxes.

- Four-year-old Maddie had severe food allergies. For most of her young life, she had a gastrointestinal tube (g-tube) placed in her abdomen so that specialized formula could be delivered directly into her stomach. Now, she was ready to learn to bite, chew, and swallow, but because she had limited experience doing so, she was not capable of eating safely. She needed an expert to guide her and her family.
- Elizabeth was referred by her pediatrician. Elizabeth, a third grader, refused to eat anything at school. She came home famished and irritable and insisted on going to a specific fast-food restaurant, where she "ate like a horse." While she maintained her growth curve for height and weight, her grades were dropping at school due to poor nutritional intake.

These were all children who needed support to continue to move forward in the developmental process of learning to eat. No two children are alike. There are many reasons why parents bring their children to feeding therapy. In fact, therapy can be helpful during any of the various stages of oral motor development in order for kids to learn to chew, swallow, and enjoy a wide variety of foods. Therapy can also help selective eaters who will not venture away from their familiar, preferred foods.

2. What does feeding therapy look like?

It starts with an evaluation. Typically conducted by a speech-language pathologist or occupational therapist specializing in feeding and swallowing difficulties in children, these evaluations can be done in a variety of settings. In a hospital setting, the evaluation may include a team of professionals, such as a gastroenterologist, psychologist, occupational therapist and/or speech-language pathologist.

3. What does treatment address?[129]

When Coach Mel evaluates a child for the first time, she always considers three major factors that influence a child's

RAISING A HEALTHY, HAPPY EATER

ability to enjoy food: (1) Physiology (which includes sensory processing); (2) Gross and fine motor skill development; and (3) The child's behavior, temperament, and family dynamics. A feeding therapist's role is to observe and identify behaviors that kids do in order to feel safe around food. In her experience, it's very rare for a child's feeding difficulties to be strictly behavioral. Turning away from the spoon, spitting, throwing food, or even demonstrating increased anxiety in the presence of new foods can be responses to poor physiology, difficulty processing sensory input, and/or inadequate motor skills. For example, a child with consistent gastrointestinal discomfort quickly learns that eating creates pain. Although the pain may be alleviated with medication, the learned behavior (e.g., fussing or refusing to sit for meals) still needs to be addressed. A feeding therapist's job is to help the child decrease anxiety and increase confidence and, slowly, improve the ability to tolerate new foods over time. Last but not least, a feeding therapist must always consider the big picture. A child's temperament and relationship with food influences the family's relationship with food and can alter family dynamics in a very unhealthy manner.

4. How long will therapy take?

Every child in feeding therapy presents with unique challenges. Length of therapy is dependent on how early in life intervention begins and the degree of medical, sensory, and behavioral needs. Typically, the therapist will assess and treat the child for two to three sessions in order to have a reasonable idea of all the factors that come into play. Some children require intensive therapy several times a day, but one session per week for about an hour is more typical. Many kids are in feeding therapy for at least one year. Occasionally, a shorter course is all a family needs to get back on the path to happier mealtimes.

5. My kid already had feeding therapy and it didn't work— how would this be different?

Please, try again, keeping in mind that perhaps a different

method of treatment is a better fit for your family. Again, no two kids are alike and a cookie-cutter approach only works if, well, you're making cookies. The best therapists are the ones that see the bigger picture and ask: "What approach is best for this child and just as importantly, this family?"[130]

6. Can't you just get him to eat a vegetable?[131]

Often, this is where parents want to start and end treatment: "If you can get him to eat broccoli, that's good enough!" A feeding therapist's job is to break each step in this complicated journey into tiny, manageable tasks that build success over time and yes, lead to healthy, nutritious eating. But if a child won't sit at the table for mealtimes or is so sensitive to aromas that just being near the kitchen causes him to gag, then there is still quite a bit of preliminary work to do before a child will chew and swallow broccoli. He'll get there, with time, but remember that the later feeding therapy starts, the more "unlearning" will need to be done. First, kids have to unlearn the behavior of running from the table or gagging. Sometimes gagging is due to sensory overload or because it is now a conditioned response to the pressure to eat. And, we can't just focus on one food, assuming that others will follow. It's more likely that the child will quickly get bored of the new vegetable and once again refuse to eat it, unless we help him to learn to taste a variety of new foods on a regular basis.

7. She eats fine at school—but at home, she won't eat what I cook. Is it my cooking?[132]

Feeding therapists consider all environments, examining why certain settings are successful and others are not. It's unlikely it's your cooking. More likely, it's a conditioned response to the environment, plus a child's expectations of what is acceptable at home versus school. A feeding therapist doesn't just focus on food. Creating positive family dynamics and adapting skills to other food environments are important to treatment. One advantage to working with a home- and community-based therapist is that feeding therapy can occur almost anywhere.

8. **Does my child have to meet with the feeding therapist? Can't you just tell me what to do?**[133]

Coach Mel explains it this way: "When a parent writes or calls me asking for help but does not want to begin one-on-one treatment, the best I can do is give general advice. A mechanic can offer general tips on how to keep your car engine running smoothly. But just like a mechanic needs to listen to the engine when it's not operating effectively, I need to observe your child and family's unique relationship with food, take a close look at your child's medical and developmental history, and then devise a plan specific to your child and family's needs. Even then, it takes a professional to adjust the process on a weekly basis."

9. **My pediatrician says my child is following a steady growth curve and will grow out of the picky eating—is that true?**[134]

While it's reassuring that he's getting enough calories to grow, are his brain and organs getting enough nutrition to be healthy and function properly? Yes, kids typically go through a picky stage in the toddler years, and some grow out of it—but some do not. If the pickiness is persisting for more than two months, seems to be getting worse, or is causing stress for your family, seeking support early on—even if for a short time to ensure that mealtimes do not become battlegrounds—may be time well spent. It's much more difficult to "unlearn" years of picky eating habits later in life.

As we've noted, parenting proactively is vital to helping kids eat. Always trust your intuition. If you suspect a feeding consult would be helpful, bring it up with your pediatrician. Your pediatrician will appreciate your perspective and willingness to have a conversation around your concerns.

10. **What's the difference between working with a nutritionist and other types of "food coaches?"**

The terms "nutritionist" and "dietitian" can be confusing. In short, all dietitians are nutritionists, but not all nutritionists are registered dietitians. When working with a specialist who focuses on nutrition, we recommend seeking help from a registered dietitian nutritionist (RDN) or a registered dietitian (RD), both credentialed through the Commission on Dietetic Registration. We are so grateful for the support of RDs and RDNs!

The difference between working with a nutritionist and either a certified speech-language pathologist (CCC-SLP) or registered occupational therapist (OTR) is that SLPs and OTRs often have specific training in the gross, fine, and oral motor skills necessary for learning to eat, as well as expert knowledge in sensory processing and medical conditions that impact a child's ability to eat. Many RDs and RDNs will suggest a feeding evaluation through an OTR or SLP just to ensure that no motor delays are contributing to the child's difficulties with food. Sometimes, the RD or RDN will collaborate with a feeding specialist who is an OTR or SLP. No matter what credentials follow a professional's name, it's important to ask the following questions, because OTRs and SLPs have a wide range of roles in their professions and may not necessarily be focused on feeding:

- How often have you treated children with feeding challenges who were diagnosed with _____? *(Fill in your child's unique medical diagnosis or special circumstances here.)* Did they make progress with you? Do you feel comfortable with your skill set treating those children?
- Tell me about your experience treating feeding challenges. How many years have you been solely focused on feeding and pediatrics?

The truth is, the term "food coach" is a general term that can apply to anyone from a personal trainer to the waiter who is helping you pick your entrée from a menu. Coach Mel, an SLP, often explains to little children that she is a food coach, much like their soccer or gymnastics coach, and that she is going to help them learn about new foods. Choosing a professional with credentials and years of feeding experience, and one who is recommended by your child's physician, is essential.

11. Where do I find help?

Your pediatrician can help connect you with the appropriate resources, including the following:

- Early-intervention services for children birth to age three. Call your local school district and ask if they have experienced therapists to evaluate your child for feeding issues. Evaluations are typically free (or low-cost) and include assessing gross and fine motor skills, speech, and more. If your child qualifies based on that evaluation, treatment is often provided for free or for very low cost regardless of income. It must be conducted in the natural environment, most often in the home or day care/preschool.
- Call your local children's hospital and request a feeding evaluation.
- Private therapists who sometimes do home visits can be found via the American Speech Language Association's "find a pro" link at asha.org. An excellent source of OTRs trained in feeding and/or sensory integration, a strong component of feeding therapy, can be found at the American Occupational Therapy Association's website, aota.org.[135]

LADIES AND GENTLEMEN, YOU'VE ARRIVED AT YOUR DESTINATION!

Raising a child comes with so many different emotions, but one thing is for sure: From the moment parents lay eyes on their baby, they know that their lives have changed. Suddenly, the sense of responsibility to nurture and raise a healthy, happy child fills the room. The enormous wave of instantaneous love— well, it's a memory that every parent has of the first time they hold their child.

We cherish our kids instinctively with our whole hearts, but it's impossible to have all the innate knowledge on how to parent when life changes daily as baby grows. Feeding a child is a complex skill that requires finesse, and the art of feeding one child can be so vastly different from feeding another. It's easy to see why we can go off course when we teach our children how to eat, no matter how good our intentions are.

As you've learned while reading *Raising a Healthy, Happy Eater*, eating first begins reflexively but in fact is a process that babies and children learn purposely over time. The way that we feed our kids influences the way they learn to eat. Outside influences, including extended family, schools, and the community contribute significantly to a child's feeding journey. Plus, if your child has feeding detours because of medical or developmental challenges, such as prematurity, sensory processing difficulties, or other physiological aspects of growth, the journey becomes even more complicated. Getting through the process takes time and patience.

But it also has its joys. This feeding adventure had to have some priceless Kodak moments! We hope you remembered to take lots of video and plenty of pictures: There was the pea puree on her little face, the fistfuls of finger foods, the messy toddler apron she wore as she helped you make granola bites, and her first lunch box packed with the wholesome food you prepared together. Even more remarkable is the journey beyond food: Do you remember the times you let go of the fear and parented bravely and joyfully? Or the moments that you took time to parent proactively and mindfully? The patience it took to parent consistently and compassionately? You've learned that these practices live so far beyond the kitchen.

By following seven important parenting strategies, you've become accustomed to how to manage the incredible responsibility of raising a happy and healthy eater. We hope that along the way, you have had a lot of fun in the kitchen and made wonderful memories with your little one—and that you continue to foster your child's love for healthy food throughout her life. There is so much joy to be had in every step.

Ladies and gentlemen, you've arrived at your destination: You have a healthy, happy eater thriving in a family culture of wellness. Maybe, on occasion, you're enjoying a bite of fast food, or maybe not. But making frequent trips to the drive-through, grabbing processed foods on the run while lost in a culture of convenience, isn't a path you travel on an everyday basis. You've established a balanced approach to feeding. You've created your own path, unique to your family, while respecting the developmental process that each child must go through in order to learn to try new foods. We personally want to thank you for the effort and the perseverance when the climb got a bit steep. Being intentional when raising a healthy, happy eater isn't always easy, but it's worth it, and we are grateful to have been a part of your family's journey.

Endnotes
· · · · · · · · · · ·

1 "How Americans Eat Today." CBS.com. January 12, 2010.
2 Eicher, Mark L. "Feeding." *Children with Disabilities*, 621–641. 4th ed. Baltimore, MD: Paul H. Brookes, 1997.
3 Arvedson, Joan C. *Pediatric Swallowing and Feeding: Assessment and Management*. San Diego, CA: Singular Pub. Group, 1993.
4 Potock, Melanie. *Happy Mealtimes with Happy Kids: How to Teach Your Child About the Joy of Food!: Practical and Surprising Tips from a Pediatric Feeding Specialist*. Longmont, CO: My Munch Bug Pub., 2010: 24.
5 Ayres, A. Jean, and Jeff Robbins. *Sensory Integration and the Child*. Los Angeles, CA: Western Psychological Services, 1979. 5–6.
6 Potock, Melanie. "Our Perception of Taste: What's Sound Got to Do with It." ASHAsphere. March 14, 2014.
7 Eplett, Layla. "Pitch/Fork: The Relationship Between Sound and Taste." *Scientific American* online. September 13, 2013.
8 Potock. "Our Perception of Taste."
9 Mouly, Anne-Marie, and Regina Sullivan. "Chapter 15: Memory and Plasticity in the Olfactory System: From Infancy to Adulthood." *The Neurobiology of Olfaction*, 1. Boca Raton, FL: CRC Press, 2010.
10 Franks, KM and JS Isaacson. "Synapse-Specific Downregulation of NMDA Receptors by Early Experience: A Critical Period for Plasticity of Sensory Input to Olfactory Cortex." *Neuron* 47 (2005): 1–14.
11 Yuhas, Daisy. "Savory Science: Jelly Bean Taste Test." *Scientific American* online.
12 Bartoshuk, LM. "Comparing Sensory Experiences Across Individuals: Recent Psychophysical Advances Illuminate Genetic Variation in Taste Perception." *Chem. Senses* 25, no. 4 (2000): 447–460.
13 Reedy, FE Jr. "Variations in Human Taste Bud Density and Taste Intensity Perception." *Physiol Behav.* 47, no. 6 (1990): 1213–1219.
14 Ventura, AK and Jeff Worobey. "Early Influences on the Development of Food Preferences." *Curr Biol.* 23, no. 9 (2013): R401–408.
15 Manella, JA. "Ontogeny of Taste Preferences." *Am J Clin Nutr.* 99, no. 3 (2014): S706–711.
16 Frazier, AL, CA Camargo Jr., Camargo S. Malspeis, WC Willet, and MC Young. "Prospective Study of Peripregnancy Consumption of Peanuts or Tree Nuts by Mothers and the Risk of Peanut or Tree Nut Allergy in Their Offspring." *JAMA Pediatr.* 168, no. 2 (2014): 156–162.

17 Bahr, Diane Chapman. *Nobody Ever Told Me (or My Mother) That!: Everything from Bottles and Breathing to Healthy Speech Development.* Arlington, TX: Sensory World, 2010. 25.

18 "Frequently Asked Questions." International Affiliation of Tongue-Tie Professionals. tonguetieprofessionals.org/faq/.

19 Bahr. *Nobody Ever Told Me (or My Mother) That!* 13.

20 Robinson, Kara. "What to Do When Baby Refuses a Bottle." WebMD. January 27, 2014.

21 "Non-nutritive Sucking." Oral Health Initiative: A Program from the American Academy of Pediatrics. http://www2.aap.org/oralhealth/pact/ch8_sect1b.cfm.

22 "Changing Concepts of Sudden Infant Death Syndrome: Implications for Infant Sleeping Environment and Sleep Position." *Pediatrics* 105, no. 3; (2000): 650–656.

23 "Belly Balls Lactation Education Tool." Breastfeeding Made Simple. breastfeedingmadesimple.com/AmedaBellyBallsCard.pdf.

24 Poyak, J. "Effects of Pacifiers on Early Oral Development." *Int J Orthod Milwaukee* 17, no. 4 (2006): 13–16.

25 American College of Obstetricians and Gynecologists. "Definition of Term Pregnancy. Committee Opinion Number 579." *Obstet Gynecol.* 122 (2013): 1139–1140.

26 Dodd, VL. "Implications of Kangaroo Care for Growth and Development in Preterm Infants." *J Obstet Gynecol Neonatal Nurs.* 34, no. 2 (2005): 218–232.

27 Potock, Melanie. "All I Want for Christmas Is My G-Tube Out!" ASHAsphere. December 5, 2013.

28 Bahr. *Nobody Ever Told Me (or My Mother) That!* 51.

29 Potock, Melanie. "Baby Led Weaning: A Developmental Perspective." ASHAsphere. February 4, 2014.

30 Ibid.

31 Zeiger, Stacey. "Why Do Babies Respond Strongly to a Game of Peekaboo?" Mom.me.

32 Greer, FR, SH Sicherer, WA Burks, and the Committee on Nutrition and Section on Allergy and Immunology. "Effects of Early Nutritional Interventions on the Development of Atopic Disease in Infants and Children: The Role of Maternal Dietary Restriction, Breastfeeding, Timing of Introduction of Complementary Foods, and Hydrolyzed Formulas." *Pediatrics* 121, no. 1 (2008): 183–191.

33 Greene, Alan. "White Out." drgreene.com.

34 Potock. *Happy Mealtimes with Happy Kids: How to Teach Your Child About the Joy of Food!* 1–5.

35 Pepper, Jan, and Elaine Weitzman. *It Takes Two to Talk: A Practical Guide for Parents of Children with Language Delays.* 3rd ed. Toronto: Hanen Centre, 2004.

36 Longtin, Susan, and Sima Gerber. "Contemporary Perspectives on Facilitating Language Acquisition for Children on the Autistic Spectrum: Engaging the Parent and the Child." floortime.org.

37 Ovsenik, Melanie. "Incorrect Orofacial Functions Until 5 Years of Age and Their Association with Posterior Crossbite." *Am J Orthod Dentofacial Orthop* 136, no. 6 (2009): 375–381.

38 Keim, SA, EN Fletcher, MR TePoel, and LB McKenzie. "Injuries Associated with

Bottles, Pacifiers, and Sippy Cups in the United States, 1991–2010." 129, no. 6 (2012): 1104–1110.

39   Marshalla, Pam. *How to Stop Thumbsucking and Other Oral Habits: Practical Solutions for Home and Therapy*. Kirkland, WA: Marshalla Speech and Language, 2001. 22.

40   Coulthard, H., G. Harris, and P. Emmett. "Delayed Introduction of Lumpy Foods to Children During the Complementary Feeding Period Affects Child's Food Acceptance and Feeding at 7 Years of Age." *Matern Child Nutr.* 5, no. 1 (2009): 75–85.

41   Potock, Melanie. "You Want My Kid to Play in Food? Seriously?" ASHAsphere. September 25, 2014.

42   Ibid.

43   Ibid.

44   Kearney, Albert J. *Understanding Applied Behavior Analysis: an Introduction to ABA for Parents, Teachers, and Other Professionals*. London: Jessica Kingsley Publishers, 2008: 20.

45   "Feeding and Swallowing Disorders (Dysphagia) in Children." American Speech-Language-Hearing Association.

46   Potock, Melanie. "Pediatric Feeding Case Study: Zachary – Age 3:11." PediaStaff. July 26, 2011.

47   Yoda, *The Empire Strikes Back*. Directed by Irvin Kershner, Twentieth Century Fox, 1980.

48   Droit-Volet, S., and S. Rousset. "How Emotions Expressed by Adults' Faces Affect the Desire to Eat Liked and Disliked Foods in Children Compared to Adults." *British Journal of Developmental Psychology* 30, no. 2 (2012): 253–266.

49   Fernando, Nimali. "Taste Testing Fun from Doctor Yum." karenlebBillon.com. June 6, 2014.

50   Potock, Melanie. "Preventing Food Jags: What's a Parent to Do?" ASHAsphere. June 12, 2014.

51   Ibid.

52   Klara, R. "Table the Issue. The Elements That Make up a Tabletop Can Be Very Important. But Do Customers Really Notice Them?" *Restaurant Business* 103, no. 18 (2004): 14–15.

53   Wansink, B., K. Van Ittersum, and JE Painter. "Ice Cream Illusions Bowls: Spoons, and Self-served Portion." *American Journal of Preventive Medicine* 31, no. 3 (2006): 240–243.

54   Rolls, BJ, DL Engell, and LL Birch. "Serving Portion Size Influences 5-year-old but Not 3-year-old Children's Food Intakes." *J Am Diet Assoc* 100, no. 2 (2000): 232–234.

55   "Food Scores." Environmental Working Group. ewg.org/foodscores#.

56   Norman, Joshua. "Fast Food Chains Target Babies: Study." cbsnews.com/news/fast-food-chains-target-babies-study.

57   Otten JJ. *Food Marketing: Using Toys to Market Children's Meals*. Minneapolis, MN: Healthy Eating Research; 2014. Available at healthyeatingresearch.org.

58   Merlo, LJ, C. Klingman, TH Malasanos, and JH Silverstein. "Exploration of Food Addiction in Pediatric Patients: A Preliminary Investigation." *J Addict Med* 3, no. 1 (2009): 26–32.

59   Avena, NM, R. Rada, and BG Hoebel. "Evidence for Sugar Addiction: Behavioral and Neurochemical Effects of Intermittent, Excessive Sugar Intake." *Neurosci Biobehav Rev* 32, no. 1 (2008): 20–39.

60   Potock, Melanie. "Three Reasons Why Kids Get Hooked on 'Kids' Meals' . . . and How to Change That." ASHAsphere. July 3, 2013.

61   DeShazo, RD, S. Bigler, and LB Skipworth. "The Autopsy of Chicken Nuggets Reads 'Chicken Little.'" *Am J Med* 126, no. 11 (2013): 1018–1019.

62   Potock. "Three Reasons Why Kids Get Hooked on 'Kids' Meals'."

63   Ibid.

64   Ibid.

65   Ibid.

66   Ibid.

67   Le Billon, Karen. *French Kids Eat Everything: How Our Family Moved to France, Cured Picky Eating, Banished Snacking, and Discovered 10 Simple Rules for Raising Healthy, Happy Eaters.* New York: William Morrow, 2012. 209.

68   Castle, Jill, and Maryann Jacobsen. *Fearless Feeding: How to Raise Healthy Eaters from High Chair to High School.* 152.

69   Potock, Melanie. *Happy Mealtimes with Happy Kids: How to Teach Your Child about the Joy of Food!: Practical and Surprising Tips from a Pediatric Feeding Specialist.* Longmont, CO: My Munch Bug Pub., 2010. 68–70

70   Ibid. 72–73.

71   Ibid.

72   Stevens, LJ, T. Kuczek, JR Burgess, E. Hurt, and LE Arnold. "Dietary Sensitivities and ADHD Symptoms: Thirty-five Years of Research." *Clin Pediatr (Phila)* 50, no. 4 (2011): 279–293.

73   Stevens, LJ, JR Kuczek, MA Stochelski, and T. Kuczek. "Amounts of Artificial Food Dyes and Added Sugars in Foods and Sweets Commonly Consumed by Children." *Clin Pediatr (Phila)* 54, no. 4 (2015): 309–321.

74   Lui, Jan, WT Hwang, B. Dikerman, and C. Compher. "Regular Breakfast Consumption Is Associated with Increased IQ in Kindergarten Children." *Early Hum Dev* 89, no. 4 (2013): 257–262.

75   Potock, Melanie. "What Type of Parent Are You at the Dinner Table?" dr.greene.com. February 20, 2014.

76   Ibid.

77   Baumrind, D. "Effects of Authoritative Parental Control on Child Behavior." *Child Development* 37, no. 4 (1966): 887–907.

78   Potock. "What Type of Parent Are You at the Dinner Table."

79   Ibid.

80   Ibid.

81   Blair, Dorothy. "The Child in the Garden: An Evaluative Review of the Benefits of School Gardening." *The Journal of Environmental Education* 40, no. 3 (2009): 15–38.

82   Fernando, Nimali. "And Now Let's Get the Garden Growing!" drgreene.com. February 27, 2014.

83   Committee on Nutrition and the Council on Sports Medicine and Fitness. "Sports Drinks and Energy Drinks for Children and Adolescents: Are They Appropriate?" *Pediatrics* 127, no. 8 (2011): 1182–1189.

84   Yale Rudd Center for Food Policy and Obesity. "Fast Food FACTS 2013: Measuring Progress in Nutrition and Marketing to Children and Teens." fastfoodmarketing.org. November 1, 2013. fastfoodmarketing.org/media/FastFoodFACTS_Report.pdf.

85   Stitt, C., and D. Kunkel. "Food Advertising During Children's Television Programming on Broadcast and Cable Channels." *Health Commun* 23, no. 6 (2008): 573–584.

86   Robinson, TN, DL Borzekowski, DM Matheson, and HC Kraemer. "Effects of Fast Food Branding on Young Children's Taste Preferences." *Arch Pediatr Adolesc Med* 161, no. 8 (2007): 972–977.

87   Lipsky, LM, and RJ Iannotti. "Associations of Television Viewing with Eating Behaviors in the 2009 Health Behaviour in School-aged Children Study." *Arch Pediatr Adolesc Med* 166, no. 5 (2012): 465–472.

88   Harris, JL, JA Bargh, and KD Brownell. "Priming Effects of Television Food Advertising on Eating Behavior." *Health Psychol* 28, no. 4 (2009): 404–413.

89   Council on Communications and Media. "From the American Academy of Pediatrics Policy Statement: Children, Adolescents, and the Media." *Pediatrics* 132, no. 5 (2013): 958–961.

90   Dennison, BA, TA Erb, and PL Jenkins. "Television Viewing and Television in Bedroom Associated with Overweight Risk Among Low-income Preschool Children." *Pediatrics* 109, no. 6 (2002): 1028–1035.

91   Barr-Anderson, DJ, P. Van Den Berg, D. Neumark-Sztainer, and M. Story. "Characteristics Associated with Older Adolescents Who Have a Television in Their Bedrooms." *Pediatrics* 121, no. 4 (2008): 718–724.

92   Barros, RM, EJ Silver, and RE Stein. "School Recess and Group Classroom Behavior."*Pediatrics* 123, no. 2 (2009): 431–436.

93   National Association of Early Childhood Specialists in State Departments of Education. *Recess and the Importance of Play: A Position Statement on Young Children and Recess*. Urbana, IL: National Association of Early Childhood Specialists in State Departments of Education, 2001. Retrieved from eric.ed.gov.

94   Pontifex, MB, BJ Saliba, LB Raine, DL Picchietti, and CH Hillman. "Exercise Improves Behavioral, Neurocognitive, and Scholastic Performance in Children with Attention-Deficit/Hyperactivity Disorder." *J Pediatr* 162, no. 3 (2013): 534–531.

95   Potock, Melanie. "Picky Eating at Lunch." drgreene.com. April 10, 2013.

96   Organisation for Economic Co-operation and Development. "Obesity Update." OECD. June 1, 2014. oecd.org.

97   Miller, Jon. "As Diets Change in Greece, Obesity Becomes Growing Problem." PBS News Hour. October 29, 2012.

98   Potock, Melanie. "Chaos in the School Cafeteria: How to Find the Calm." easylunchboxes.com. November 7, 2011.

99   Ibid., and Potock, Melanie. "The School Cafeteria: Hurry Up and EAT!" ASHAsphere. August 22, 2013.

100 Potock. "The School Cafeteria: Hurry Up and EAT!"

101 Ibid.

102 Ibid.

103 Potock, Melanie. "Summertime Prep for the School Cafeteria." ASHAsphere. June 13, 2013.

104 Ibid.

105 Potock, Melanie. "She Didn't Eat a Thing at School Today!" ASHAsphere. August 24, 2014.

106 Ibid.

107 Potock. "The School Cafeteria: Hurry Up and EAT!"

108 Ibid.

109 Ibid.

110 Potock, Melanie. "A Creative Approach to Food Allergies and Trick-or-Treating." ASHAsphere. October 13, 2013.

111 Ibid.

112 Ibid.

113 Lite, Lori. "Halloween Tips to Avoid Meltdowns!" Stress Free Kids. October 11, 2011.

114 Potock. "A Creative Approach to Food Allergies and Trick-or-Treating."

115 Potock, Melanie. "Tips To Help Your Food Allergic Child 'Belong' During The Holidays." Tender Foodies. November 16, 2011.

116 Potock, Melanie. "Planning for Holiday Meals with a Picky Eater." ASHAsphere. November 7, 2013.

117 Smith, Aimee. "Aimee's Story: Second Thoughts About Thanksgiving." Tender Foodie. November 10, 2011.

118 Mayo Clinic Staff. "Eosinophilic Esophagitis." June 19, 2014. mayoclinic.org

119 American Partnership for Eosinophil Disorders. "Eosinophil Associated Disorders Fact Sheet." June 1, 2011. apfed.org.

120 Food Allergy Research and Education. "About Food Allergies." foodallergy.org.

121 "Type 1 Diabetes Facts." jdrf.org.

122 Eicher. "Feeding."

123 "Autism Spectrum Disorder Data and Statistics." Centers for Disease Control and Prevention. March 24, 2014. cdc.gov.

124 Potock, Melanie. "5 Signs That Your Infant May Benefit from Feeding Therapy." Friendship Circle. February 3, 2013.

125 Ibid.

126 Ibid.

127 Potock. *Happy Mealtimes with Happy Kids*. 107.

128 Potock, Melanie. "Nine Common Questions About Feeding Therapy." generationrescue.org. February 11, 2014.

129 Ibid.

130 Ibid.

131 Ibid.

132 Ibid.

133 Ibid.

134 Ibid.

135 Potock, Melanie. "10 Things You Should Know About Feeding Therapy." Friendship Circle. January 22, 2013.

Resources:
Information and Support

ALLERGIES AND MEDICAL CONDITIONS

apfed.org (American Partnership for Eosinophilic Disorders)
foodallergy.org
jdrf.org (Type 1 diabetes)
keeleymcguire.com
nonutsmomsgroup.weebly.com
snacksafely.com
thetenderfoodie.com

CHILDREN'S HEALTH AND FEEDING

parentinginthekitchen.com (Parenting in the Kitchen with Doctor Yum and Coach Mel)
doctoryum.org (Doctor Yum's website)
mymunchbug.com (Coach Mel's website)
ewg.org
healthychildren.org

COOKING

100daysofrealfood.com
thegoodfoodfactory.com
superhealthykids.com
weelicious.com

FEEDING KIDS

Baby-led Weaning: The Essential Guide to Introducing Solid Foods
Gill Rapley and Tracey Murkett (The Experiment Publishing, 2010)
Child of Mine: Feeding with Love and Good Sense, revised edition
Ellyn Satter (Bull Publishing Company, 2000)
Colic Solved: The Essential Guide to Infant Reflux and the Care of Your Crying, Difficult-to- Soothe Baby
Bryan Vartabedian, MD (Ballantine Books, 2007)

Cure Your Child with Food
  Kelly Dorfman, MS, LND (Workman Publishing Company, 2013)
Fearless Feeding: How to Raise Healthy Eaters from High Chair to High School
  Jill Castle, MS, RD, LDN and Maryann Jacobsen, MS, RD (Jossey-Bass, 2013)
Feeding Baby Greene: The Earth Friendly Program for Healthy, Safe Nutrition During Pregnancy, Childhood, and Beyond
  Alan Greene, MD (Jossey-Bass, 2009)
Food Fights: Winning the Nutritional Challenges of Parenthood Armed with Insight, Humor and a Bottle of Ketchup
  Laura A. Jana, MD and Jennifer Shu, MD (American Academy of Pediatrics, 2012)
French Kids Eat Everything: How Our Family Moved to France, Cured Picky Eating, Banned Snacking, and Discovered 10 Simple Rules for Raising Happy, Healthy Eaters
  Karen Le Billon (William Morrow, 2014)
Getting to YUM: The 7 Secrets of Raising Eager Eaters
  Karen Le Billon (William Morrow, 2014)
Happy Mealtimes with Happy Kids: How to Teach Your Child about the Joy of Food!
  Melanie Potock, MA, CCC-SLP (My Munch Bug Publishing, 2014)
Nobody Ever Told Me (or my mother) THAT!: Everything from Bottles and Breathing to Healthy Speech Development
  Diane Bahr, MS, CCC-SLP (Sensory World, 2010)
Secrets of Feeding a Healthy Family: How to Eat, How to Raise Good Eaters, How to Cook, second edition
  Ellyn Satter, MS, RDN, MSSW (Kelcy Press, 2008)

FUN FOR KIDS
Broc and Cara's Picnic Party
  Dave Wilson (Dave Wilson Publishing, 2014)
Eating the Alphabet: Fruits & Vegetables from A to Z
  Lois Ehlert (HMH Books for Young Readers, 1993)
Food Play
  Joost Elffers and Saxton Freymann (Chronicle Books, 2006)
Recipes for Play: Creative Activities for Small Hands and Big Imaginations
  Rachel Sumner and Ruth Mitchener (The Experiment Publishing, 2014)
supersprowtz.com
zisboombah.com

GARDENING
All New Square Foot Gardening, Second Edition: The Revolutionary Way to Grow More In Less Space
  Mel Bartholomew (Cool Springs Press, 2013)

Rocks, Dirt, Worms & Weeds: A Fun, User-Friendly, Illustrated Guide to Creating a Vegetable or Flower Garden with Your Kids
Jeff Hutton (Skyhorse Publishing, 2012)

MUSIC
Dancing in the Kitchen: Songs That Celebrate the Joy of Food! at mymunchbug.com

PARENTING
Ask Supernanny: What Every Parent Wants to Know
Jo Frost (Hyperion, 2006)
Healthy Sleep Habits, Happy Child: A Step-By-Step Programme for a Good Night's Sleep
Marc Weissbluth, MD (Vermilion, 2005)
If I Have to Tell You One More Time...The Revolutionary Program That Gets Your Kids to Listen Without Nagging, Reminding, or Yelling
Amy McCready (Tarcher, 2012)
The Happiest Toddler on the Block, revised edition
Harvey Karp, MD (Bantam, 2008)
Unconditional Parenting: Moving from Rewards and Punishments to Love and Reason
Alphie Kohn (Atria Books, 2006)

PRODUCTS
arktherapeutic.com
babydipper.com
copy-kids.com
easylunchboxes.com
ezpzfun.com
funbites.com
kidcompanions.com
littlepartners.com
mymunchbug.com
numnumdips.com
superduper.com
talktools.com
todayiatearainbow.com
us.kuhnrikon.com
wubbanub.com
yumboxlunch.com

PROFESSIONAL ASSOCIATIONS
American Academy of Pediatrics, www.aap.org
American Occupational Therapy Association, www.aota.org
American Physical Therapy Association, www.apta.org
American Speech Language Hearing Asosociation, www.asha.org

International Association of Orofacial Myology, www.iaom.com
International Lactation Consultant Association, www.ilca.org

RECIPES

Bébé Gourmet: 100 French-Inspired Baby Food Recipes For Raising an Adventurous Eater
Jenny Carenco and Dr. Jean Lalau Keraly (The Experiment Publishing, 2013)

Cooking for Baby: Wholesome, Homemade, Delicious Foods for 6 to 18 Months
Lisa Barnes (Touchstone, 2009)

Cooking with Trader Joe's Cookbook: Easy Lunch Boxes
Kelly Lester (Brown Bag Publishers LLC, 2012)

Forks Over Knives The Cookbook: Over 300 Recipes for Plant-Based Eating All Through the Year
Del Sroufe and Isa Chandra Moskowitz (The Experiment Publishing, 2012)

Gluten-Free Family Favorites: The 75 Go-To Recipes You Need to Feed Kids and Adults All Day, Every Day
Kelli Bronski and Peter Bronski (The Experiment Publishing, 2014)

Learning to Bake Allergen-Free: A Crash Course for Busy Parents on Baking without Wheat, Gluten, Dairy, Eggs, Soy or Nuts
Colette Martin (The Experiment Publishing, 2012)

Mom and Me Cookbook
Annabel Karmel (DK Children, 2005)

Salad People and More Real Recipes
Molly Katzen (Tricycle Press, 2005)

SENSORY PROCESSING

Raising a Sensory Smart Child: The Definitive Handbook for Helping Your Child with Sensory Processing Issues
Lindsey Biel, OTR/L and Nancy Peske (Penguin Books, 2009)

Sensational Kids: Hope and Help for Children with Sensory Processing Disorder
Lucy Jane Miller, Ph.D., OTR (Perigee Books, 2014)

Sensory Processing Challenges: Effective Clinical Work with Kids & Teens
Lindsey Biel, OTR/L (W. W. Norton & Company, 2014)

SCHOOL AND FOOD

letsmove.gov
school-bites.com
thelunchbox.org

Photograph Credits

Photographs on pages 30, 37, 46, 50, 77, 111, 117, 126, 127, 155, 159, 178, 194, 195, 212, and 213 are courtesy of the authors.

CHAPTER 3

    page 34 courtesy of Sandra Coulson, MS, ST, Ed, COM

CHAPTER 5

    page 81 courtesy of Sandra Coulson, MS, ST, Ed, COM
    page 83 courtesy of ArkTherapeutic.com
    page 97 photo credit Sandra Sieminski
    page 102 photo credit Neville Fernando

CHAPTER 6

    page 115 drawing by Ashleigh Buyers
    page 122 courtesy of Little Partners

CHAPTER 7

    page 140 drawing by Ashleigh Buyers

Acknowledgments

Our sincere thanks—

To the team at The Experiment Publishing for understanding our intention and rooting us on every step of the way.

For Ashleigh Buyer's illustrations and graphics that have brought this book to life. From the early days of the Doctor Yum Project she has brilliantly captured the joyful spirit of feeding kids.

To Dr. Roshini Raj, who was so open to our ideas and willing to write the foreword for this book.

The "What Kids Eat Around the World" sections gave us the opportunity to connect with our worldly friends: Dr. Joanne Bassali, Nilashee Perera, and Dr. Pam Nguyen.

To the many, many professionals who offered tips and encouragement, especially Lindsey Biel, OTR/L and Diane Bahr, MS, CCC-SLP.

To the beautiful children who capture the essence of joyful eating: Abigail, Anna, Maya, Jackson, Owen, Payton, Sophie, and your wonderful parents, too!

To the parents and their children who took the time to share their emotional stories with the hope of helping others: Aimee and Raina, Erin and Gavin, Keeley and "Little Miss," Julie Kay and Jonathan, Benjamin and Gabriel.

ACKNOWLEDGMENTS

To our patients and clients who taught us the lessons we share in this book—and remind us to parent joyfully, compassionately, bravely, patiently, proactively, consistently, and mindfully.

And, with most loving gratitude, to our families, who cooked dinners and fed us, who read and reread chapter after chapter (giving their most honest opinions) and put up the Christmas tree because we were still busy writing.

Index